Preventative Medicine and Management for the Horse

Preventative Medicine and Management for the Horse

Sheridan Lee Cernik

South Brunswick and New York: A. S. Barnes and Company
London: Thomas Yoseloff Ltd

© 1977 by A. S. Barnes and Co., Inc.

A. S. Barnes and Co., Inc.
Cranbury, New Jersey 08512

Thomas Yoseloff Ltd
Magdalen House
136-148 Tooley Street
London SE1 2TT, England

Library of Congress Cataloging in Publication Data

Cernik, Sheridan Lee, 1942-
   Preventative medicine and management for the horse.

   Includes index.
   1. Horses—Diseases.   2. Horses.   I. Title.
SF951.C47   636.1′08′9   76-50192
ISBN 0-498-01925-X

This book is dedicated to
Britt and Kirsten

*In the hope that they will
someday understand the kindness
of Krishna and Hawkeye and those
horses to follow . . .*

Contents

Foreword

Horses are one of the noblest creatures on earth. They have served and continue to serve mankind in many capacities. In the early days prior to the development of mechanical horsepower, horses literally fed the nation and also provided much pleasure for man. Today in the United States, the horse provides much more pleasure than formerly, and in general, is owned and cared for in more urban than farm-type surroundings. In many cases, this causes the horse problems because he is entirely dependent on man for care and feed.

Most horse owners desire the best care for the horse, but often, because of ignorance and "old wives' tales" the horse suffers. For example, the practice of deworming the horse only in the spring and the fall was probably adequate when the horse had hundreds of acres to pasture on, thereby diminishing his chances of reinfesting himself with worms. Unfortunately, this routine is still advocated and followed by many horseowners, even though their horses are provided a very small lot to spend their lifetime in. Under these conditions, internal parasites (especially strongyle worms) needlessly harm and kill thousands of horses each year.

Many other examples of ignorance could be mentioned, but the author has done a remarkable job in updating health care and management practice information for the horse owner and caretaker.

She has adequately illustrated the text and clearly explained many of the common problems encountered in taking care of the horse. Prevention of problems has been stressed and rightly so, because our noble animal, the horse, should be cared for with the most up-to-date information available to prevent illness and injuries.

I'm sure my opinion will be shared by all readers who enjoy the horse, be it for work or pleasure.

T.N. Phillips, D.V.M.
Illinois Equine Hospital & Clinic
Naperville, Illinois

Acknowledgments

I'd like to give a very special thank you to those family members, friends, horsepeople, veterinarians, and corporations who gave unselfishly of their time and knowledge to get this book together. Much of the credit for the factuality and destruction of old equine myths goes to Dr. Thomas Phillips, my editor and friend, and Dr. Joseph Foerner of the Illinois Equine Clinic and Hospital.

To Bob Doonan and Dr. William McMullan of Texas A&M, a thank you for the help in selecting many appropriate photographs and medical information. Among the many others who helped are front cover photographer Tobe Cogswell of Farnam Companies, Inc.; Shell Chemical Co.; Dr. Cheryl Knobloch of the University of Illinois; John Ewing Company; USDA; 3M Company; Franz Studios; Cut-Heal, Inc.; Butler Manufacturing Co.; Merck & Co., Inc.; American Trakehner Association, Inc.; TPC Products; The American Humane Assoc.; Wood Products Co.; The American Paint Horse Assoc.; Stoddard Manufacturing Co.; American Quarter Horse Assoc.; Joseph Trhlik; Dr. Ronald Camden; Dr. W. J. Monson of Borden Chemical Company's Nutritional Research Lab.; Ralston Purina Co.; The Paoli Insurance Agency, Inc.; North West Rubber Mats Ltd.; and the American Veterinary Medical Association.

Preventative Medicine and Management for the Horse

1

Anatomy and Conformation

A horseperson lives with two objectives in mind, to obtain maximum performance, and maintain health and soundness of his horse. In your pursuit of serviceability from your horse, have you considered the relationship between equine health and the way the horse is put together anatomically?

There is a direct correlation, and you play a key role in maintaining the delicate balance between the two. A horse is like an intricately designed machine. Each movement is the result of coordinated interaction among bone, cartilage, tendon, muscle, ligament, tissue, and mind. If any one of the parts is weak, or structurally defective, that part, and the tissues surrounding it are vulnerable to stress. The by-products of too much stress are injury and disease—both of which quickly take your horse out of service.

If you take the time to familiarize yourself with normal and abnormal conformation—the way the horse is put together—and understand a few anatomical points, you should find it easier to comprehend how your work and management practices can stress a weak site. Then, hopefully, you'll be able to prevent a good majority of needless injuries and diseases to that area.

Bones, Joints, and Tissues

Until the horse is about five years old, his bones grow in length and circumference. During this period the young equine can be permanently damaged by poor nutritional practices, improper shoeing, disease and injury, and from work excess and poor management.

15

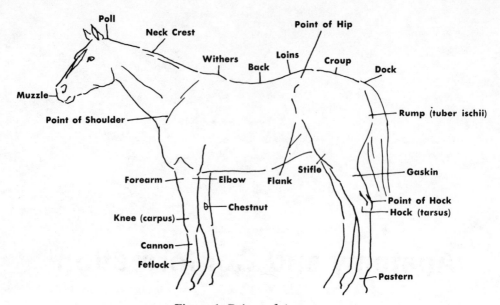

Figure 1. Points of Anatomy

In the immature horse, growth in bone length occurs at each end. The ends, themselves, are separated from the main shaft by a thin layer of cartilage. The function of this cartilage is to produce new bone cells until maturity, when hardening occurs and the ends fuse to the shaft. When all the skeletal bones are fused, the horse is at its peak strength to support your weight and riding demands.

Increase in circumference is accomplished by a two-layered tissue covering around the bone called the *periosteum* (peri, around + osteum, bone). When this membrane ceases bone cell production at maturity, its inner layer hardens. The outer layer, however, remains active and is instrumental in healing a break by manufacturing new bone cells.

A *joint*, or articulation, is formed where the bone ends fit together (Fig. 2). Joints take the major brunt of work concussion and are thus one of the major sites of lameness and soreness problems. Over the bone ends is a thin cartilage covering that makes movement easy and guards against irritation from rubbing. This cartilage is regularly "oiled" by a joint fluid known as *synovia* and manufactured by the joint capsule membrane. Besides producing synovia, the membrane, which surrounds the joint, also serves as a shock buffer when the joint area receives a blow. Additional, thicker cartilage is found as pads between the bones, and also around bone ends to cushion the shock of the bones coming together, and to produce a tighter fit where it rims the joint.

Ligaments, tendons, and muscles hold the joint together and give it movement. The *ligament* is a fibrous tissue band that has three functions: (1) to hold one bone to another, (2) to minimize vibration at the joint

16

site, and (3) to prevent muscle fatigue by helping support the joint. The *tendon* is also a fibrous band, but it connects muscle to the bone or other tissue, rather than strictly bone-to-bone, as does the ligament.

A *muscle* is a tissue designed to contract and relax to move the bones in a specific manner. Muscles usually come in sets of two, with opposing functions. In the front leg, for example, you can see the *flexor* and *extensor muscles* at work when the horse bends his leg up toward the abdomen, then straightens it (Fig. 4). The flexors contract to raise and bend the leg, and the extensors contract to lower it.

In addition to this set of muscles, there is another set, the *abductor* and *adductor muscles*, which allow side-to-side movement. Again using the leg as an example, imagine the first outward step of a two-track movement. The abductor (ab, away) muscles contract to move the leg away from the body. When the leg is moved toward the body, the abductor muscles relax and the adductor (ad, toward) muscles contract. Thus, the alternate con-

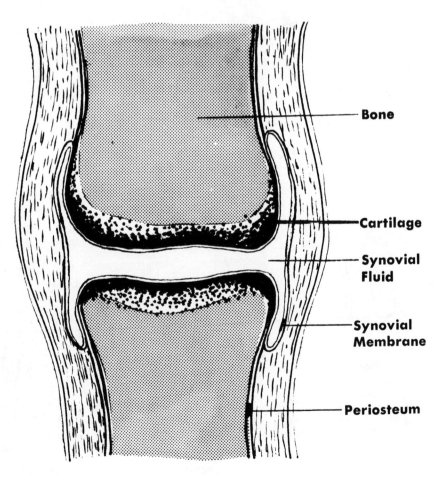

Figure 2. Synovial Joint

17

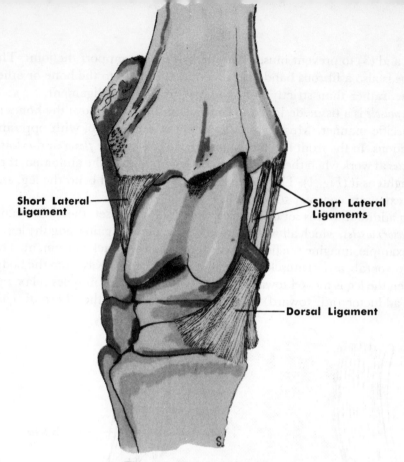

Short Lateral Ligament

Short Lateral Ligaments

Dorsal Ligament

Figure 3. Right Hock Joint

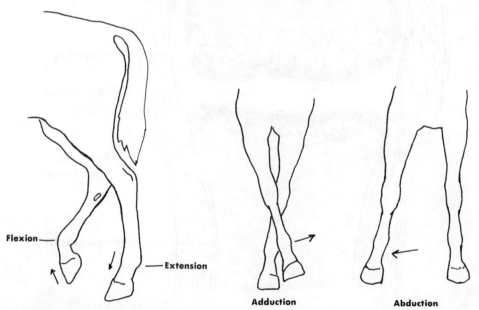

Flexion

Extension

Adduction

Abduction

Figure 4. Patterns of muscle sets.

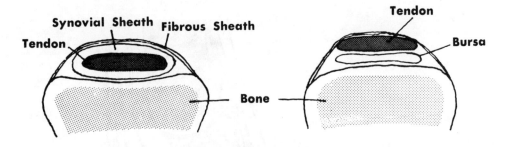

Figure 5. The synovial sheath and the bursa are protective cushions for the tendon.

traction and relaxation of sets of muscles affords an infinite variety of movements.

At certain points of the anatomy are irritation sites, caused by parts moving over or against other parts. To protect these sensitive tissues from rubbing and damage, nature developed wraps and cushionlike devices to minimize friction. The tendon is wrapped in a synovia-filled sleeve, called a *synovial sheath*, when it's long enough to travel long distances over limb parts. There's also a synovia-filled pouch, called the *bursa*, at irritation points where a joint meets a tendon, ligament, or skin. The bursa doubles as a shock absorber for blows and pressure in sites like the point of the elbow or hock, and the front of the knee.

Attention has been given to explaining basic anatomy so when you read about forthcoming diseases and injuries, you'll be able to recognize the site, and more easily understand why the specific problem developed.

The Foot

The foot is one of the most important anatomical parts of the horse. It carries out four important functions: (1) supports immense body weight, (2) helps circulate blood throughout the internal foot, (3) acts as a major shock absorber, and (4) protects sensitive internal parts from excessive concussion. The foot has an immense responsibility for such a proportionately small part of the horse's total body weight and size. Thus, if severely or permanently damaged, the result is similar to a tire blowout. Only on the equine vehicle, you don't have a spare in the trunk.

Look at Figure 6, and you'll see how the foot is designed to expand to spare the inside sensitive structures from excess shock. The dense, but elastic *hoof wall* is somewhat A-shaped to allow expansion at the base. At the back of the foot, the fleshy *heel bulbs* are minus a heavy wall so they, too, can spread when the foot touches the ground.

Below the hairline, the hard wall begins as an inch-wide strip of tough tissue called the *coronary band* or *coronet*. Hoof cells are produced in a groove

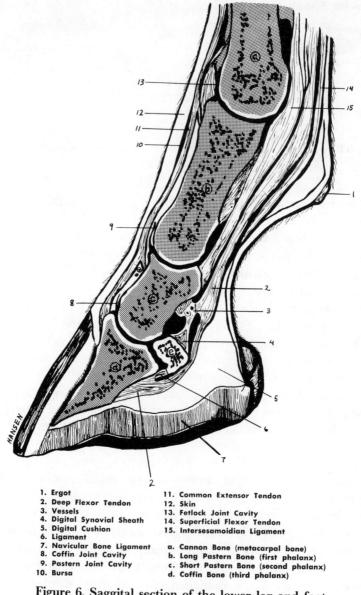

Figure 6. Saggital section of the lower leg and foot.

1. Ergot
2. Deep Flexor Tendon
3. Vessels
4. Digital Synovial Sheath
5. Digital Cushion
6. Ligament
7. Navicular Bone Ligament
8. Coffin Joint Cavity
9. Pastern Joint Cavity
10. Bursa
11. Common Extensor Tendon
12. Skin
13. Fetlock Joint Cavity
14. Superficial Flexor Tendon
15. Intersesamoidian Ligament

a. Cannon Bone (metacarpal bone)
b. Long Pastern Bone (first phalanx)
c. Short Pastern Bone (second phalanx)
d. Coffin Bone (third phalanx)

under the band and grow down at the rate of about three-eighths of an inch per month. The wall, itself, is composed of three insensitive layers: (1) the shiny outer layer or periople, (2) middle layer, and (3) the inner or insensitive laminary layer.

The *periople* functions as a varnish-like coating to keep moisture in the foot. If you remove this layer by rasping or sanding, the foot dries out, loses elasticity, and eventually cracks. The *middle layer* is quite dense, pigmented, and thicker at the toe than at the heels. It's composed of some six hundred tiny springs running from the band to the ground surface, rather like little pogo sticks. The purpose of this construction is to allow for longitudinal compression and expansion of the outer wall.

Further into the hoof is found the last layer of the hoof wall. The *insensitive laminary layer* is formed from about five hundred small, longitudinal laminae that resemble a pleated lampshade. Like the tubules of the middle layer, the insensitive laminae of the inner layer also facilitate wall expansion, but by opening out, not by compressing and expanding.

Pick up the foot and on the ground surface you'll find the insensitive structures called the bars, frog, and sole. The hoof wall is seen as a semi-circular shape around the front and sides of the foot and ends at the back with two, inward-curved, weight-bearing *bars*. These are hard supports for the rear of the foot, and lie on either side of the frog.

The composition of the *frog* is about fifty percent water, so it's relatively soft and elastic, though insensitive on the outside. With the aid of its central and side grooves (sulci or furrows), the frog functions like a tire tread. It establishes secure ground contact, while flattening and expanding to absorb shock and squeeze blood from the foot.

Unlike the frog and bars, which touch the ground, the adjacent *sole* bruises easily and is concave in design to avoid most ground pressure. It does lower slightly when the weight of the horse pushes down the internal structures on top of it.

Now we proceed from the external, insensitive structures toward the inner, sensitive structures of the foot. All sensitive parts begin where the insensitive laminary layer meshes with the *sensitive laminary layer* of the internal foot. If you look at the ground surface of a newly trimmed foot, you can see the semicircular *white line* or *quick*. This is formed at the point where the two laminary layers mesh firmly together. The sensitive laminae attach to the periosteum covering the *coffin bone,* and to the *lateral cartilages* on either side of the bone. This bond ensures a firm union of the outside hoof wall with the internal parts.

The coffin bone is lightweight, porous, and rich in blood vessels. At its upper front surface is a projection called the *extensor process.* It serves as an attachment site for the common extensor muscle tendon. Lying between the coffin bone's two, long, posterior extensions is the *navicular bone* or *distal sesamoid,* which functions as a fulcrum to stabilize the overlying flexor tendon. This tendon attaches to the underside of the coffin bone and runs up the back of the leg.

On either side of the coffin bone are elastic lateral cartilages to protect it and aid in pushing out the sides of the walls. You can easily feel the tops of these winglike structures above the coronary band. Each cartilage is aided in expansion by an elastic, fibrous pad, the *digital cushion,* lying under the coffin bone. It absorbs downward shock, and flattens to push the cartilages out and the frog down when the foot hits the ground.

A lot of emphasis has been placed on *wall expansion* because it's the salvation of the entire foot. If the wall remained rigid when the foot touched the ground, the concussion would split the outer wall and bruise the tissues within. Expansion is complicated, but works something like this: the horse's foot touches the ground and his descending body weight pushes the coffin bone onto the cushion beneath. The cushion flattens down and out and the lateral cartilages bulge against the side walls. Simultaneously, the frog and sole move down and expand. All of this outward pressure opens the laminae so they can assist in expanding the circumference of the hoof.

When the ground has reached its maximum yielding point it exerts a stationary force. This force causes the frog to flatten and widen as the weight of the horse continues to bear down on the foot. The blood vessels overlying the sensitive internal portion of the frog are squeezed between the cushion and the internal frog, so the blood moves out of the area.

Finally, the wall has yielded to all pressure from within and below, and a large part of the shock is absorbed. Until the foot is lifted, all parts remain in this position. It's easy to understand how much work is done by the foot if you imagine the rapidity of this cycle when the horse is running.

EVALUATING CONFORMATION

The way in which a horse's bones and tissues are formed and assembled is called *conformation*. If the conformation is "good," it means that the animal is well conformed from standards formulated to achieve maximum use with minimum irritation. Thus, that horse is suited to handle almost any job with ease and minimum physical stress.

Good conformation is also directly related to several other important facts. These are (1) how sound he'll remain with work, (2) how his traits will pass on to offspring, (3) how functional and varied in performance he'll be, (4) how comfortable he is to ride, and (5) how many veterinarian and farrier bills you'll receive.

If you've been around horses for a while, you've probably seen a few examples of "bad" conformation. What is really meant by that ominous-sounding phrase? Based on professional judgments, the term indicates that undesirable conformation constitutes a fault that handicaps the horse in performing to his peak ability by predisposing him to injury or disease.

Faults may be slight enough to overlook if a horse otherwise hangs together well. If they're not, faults are weak sites that can deteriorate with work and put your horse out of service for a short time or forever. These weak sites can flare up once or chronically recur.

Poor conformation, unfortunately, is not only aggravated by work. There are several other aggravations—poor shoeing, improper management and nutrition practices, oversupplementing with vitamins and minerals, diseases, injuries—that take their toll.

Now you might be asking why a misalignment in two bones can cause all this trouble. Basically, it's because that deviation in joint alignment constitutes a weakened area, as already discussed. Since the site is vulnerable to concussion, stress, and strain, it will become injured or irritated if traumatized enough.

The first symptoms of a problem are usually heat and swelling in the area, and, if the leg or foot is involved, a reluctance to move out or evident lameness. In some cases, secondary complications arise with the introduction of bacteria into the area. So your veterinarian ends up treating the initial cause of the problem plus the secondary condition. When treatment is impossible, too expensive, or too lengthy to save the horse, the only recourse is to retire him from service or put him down. Hence, the importance of trying to select a horse with good leg, foot, and body conformation.

Where do you start looking at conformation? At about twenty feet away, so you can take in the total horse, still and moving. What you see should look like a total functioning unit: all parts proportionate to each other in size, circumference, and length. The relationship between body parts—such as where the head joins the neck, and where muscles tie into leg joints—should blend smoothly. Good, flowing movement in all gaits will give you a clue as to quality of conformation and comfort of the ride.

Judging conformation is a job for a trained eye. When you find a horse that is visually pleasing to you, be sure to have a veterinarian look over that animal and point out possible problem areas. Since you'll have to pay for that professional judgment, you can eliminate many ill-conformed horses yourself by learning to identify major problem areas.

Conformation Faults

Avoid a coarse-looking head attached to a short, thick neck, since this horse will probably have two additional, undesirable features: short, upright shoulders, and similarly shaped pasterns. Both of these predispose to choppy strides and a lot of concussion on the legs and the rider. Chunky, compact horses also lack a lot of the suppleness and maneuverability that make riding a pleasure and a horse easy to handle.

The withers and slope of shoulders are important conformation landmarks. If a horse does not have a well-muscled, prominent withers, he'll generally be heavy on the forehand and unable to sustain speed without tendon, muscle, and joint fatigue. As for your comfort, owning a horse with *mutton withers* will be irritating because the saddle will tend to slip, girth sores will be a problem, and the ride will generally be uncomfortable.

Next the back: avoid a *roached* (humpd) back, sway back, or overly short or long back. A roached back hinders extension and predisposes to a motion problem called *forging* (discussed later in the chapter). A very *short back* robs the gait of smoothness, speed, and extension, while adding to joint concussion. An overly *long back* is weak and inhibits attempts at collection.

LEG CONFORMATION

Lameness is a word that immediately causes a sinking feeling in your stomach when it applies to your horse, so a very close look will be taken at the conformation faults that predispose to lameness. If you're able to spot any of them in your horse or the one you wish to purchase, you can take preventative steps to drastically reduce the chance of a problem at that site. By keeping an eye on your management practices, the shoer, and your work demands, it's possible to reduce the amount of stress on a weak area. It's also a good idea to go on to the next horse, if the one you want to buy has severe faults.

The Forelegs—Front View

To help visualize the correct relationship among parts, imagine dropping a plumbline from each shoulder point. Ideally it should bisect

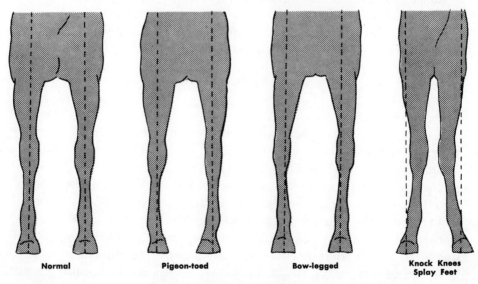

Normal   Pigeon-toed   Bow-legged   Knock Knees
                                                          Splay Feet

Figure 7. Forelimb Conformation

the leg and foot to the ground (Fig. 7). Look for the knee and fetlock joints to be proportioned to each other, and also in proportion to the size of the horse. An equal distance between the points of the shoulder and the center line through each hoof will give the horse a stable base of support. Allow about two hands width between the front legs of an adult, at chest level, and enough distance in a youngster to show promise as an adult.

Quality and size of bone are important in the cannon bone lying beneath the knee. Good bone, in cross-section, is oval, wider from side to side, and devoid of bumps. Below the cannon bone, the ankles should be of good size, and the hooves set straight ahead and equal in size and shape.

Now that you know what the "ideal" horse should look like from the front, let's take a look at the faults that can predispose to problems, depending on their severity.

1. A *wide base of support* is commonly seen in horses with weedy conformation and a narrow chest (Fig. 8). Because the horse needs a firm base

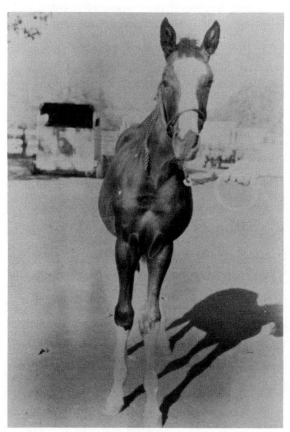

Figure 8. This is the widest base of support afforded to this foal due to his absence of chest.

of support not afforded by his narrow chest, he achieves balance by placing his legs apart, or outside the vertical plumbline. In addition, many horses also turn their toes out in a splay-footed position for more stability. Both deviations stress the *inside* of the leg.

A wide base of support causes the horse to tire easily with speed and hard work. It predisposes to articular windpuffs, ringbone of the pastern joint(s), medial splint(s), medial sidebone(s), medial fetlock joint irritation, and tendon/ligament strain.

As with the majority of conformation faults, there is no correction for this support base. There is, however, a possibility of altering any toe deviation. If this is done in one or two shoeings, or in excess, additional stress is put on the legs.

2. A *narrow support base*, with the legs deviating toward the center of the body, is usually seen in wide-chested, muscular horses. It's often accompanied by one or both toes that turn out. This combination places a strain on the *inside* aspect of the pastern, as well as the outside of the legs. The gait fault produced by a narrow base is *ambling*, a very fatigueing way of going for speed and maneuver work.

3. A *pigeon-toed* horse may turn in one or both feet (unilateral or bi-

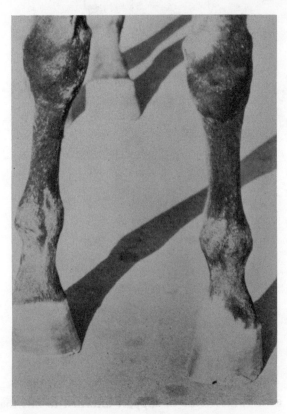

Figure 9. An extreme case of pigeon-toes.

26

lateral deviation). This problem is caused when there's an inward deviation or twisting at the shoulder joint, or as low as the fetlock joint (Fig. 9). Toeing-in is common to horses utilizing both support bases just discussed, and is a potential source of lameness due to the strain it puts on the outside (lateral) ligaments and joints of the leg. In addition to predisposing to windpuffs, pastern joint ringbone, splint(s), and sidebone(s), the defect causes a striding problem called *paddling*. Corrective trimming early in life can aid the problem, but adult correction is usually minor in value.

4. A *splay-footed* horse may turn out on one or both feet, and is generally of narrow body conformation with either base support for balance. The majority of horses that toe-out have the joint deviation occurring at the elbow level, rather than the ankle.

The strain on the inside area of the leg and foot predisposes to medial (inside) splint development and fracture, injury to the medial proximal sesamoid bone, and tendon/ligament strain. These problems are magnified in a narrow-chested horse.

Toeing-out also causes the horse to *wing* and *interfere*, two striding problems that result in additional leg injury. Splay-feet are more serious than pigeon-toes in the amount of strain they put on the legs, but some correction can be attained with proper corrective shoeing and trimming.

5. *Knock knees* develop from an inward deviation of one or both knees in adults. Affected foals usually develop this deviation because of a nutritional deficiency. The problem is not correctible in adults, but may be rectified in foals with surgical correction. Knock knees predispose to the striding defect of *interference*.

6. *Bowlegs* are the opposite of knock knees in appearance. Because the outward deviation of the knees causes the horse to stand with its weight on the outside of the feet, lateral sidebones and low ringbone frequently develop. Strain on the soft tissue and irritation of the carpal (knee) bones is also common and increases with hard work.

Bowlegs may be altered to some degree in the foal, with surgical aid, but are incurable in the adult. They predispose to *interference* when working the horse at high speeds.

7. *Bench knees*, or offset cannon bones, can occur unilaterally or bilaterally. The defect gives the area below and to the inside of the knee the appearance of having been chiseled out.

Bench knees are common and often hereditary, but are more of a developmental flaw in the young, growing foal. During the growth phase of the radius (the bone above the knee), its inside end grows more rapidly than the outside end. This causes a slight shifting of the distal end of the radius and the carpal bones to a lateral (outside), or offset position over the cannon bone.

The defect predisposes to medial splints and ligament damage re-

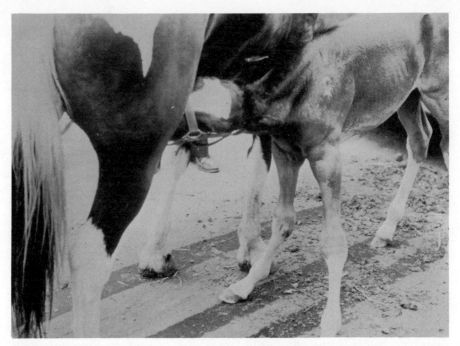

Figure 10. This foal is knock-kneed in the right fore and slightly bowed in the left foreleg.

sulting from the strain on the inside of the cannon area. The medial knee bones are also susceptible to injury and fracture. Additional complications result from numerous striding defects caused when the cannon bone is twisted at the knee joint and the toes deviate in or out.

The Forelegs—Side View

After analyzing the horse face to face, walk around to the side and look at leg conformation from that angle. Take your plumbline and mentally reposition it so it hangs from the center of the shoulder blade and bisects the side surface of the knee down to the ankle.

An ideally shaped leg will have a long, sloping shoulder coming down from prominent, muscled withers, and a muscular forearm that blends into a large, unblemished knee. The cannon bone should lie directly under the knee in a supportive position, be dense of bone, and not as long as the forearm radius. A well-conformed pastern is of moderate length, and blends into the hoof on the same sloping plane.

The faults (Fig. 11) to look for from the side view are:

1. The *upright shoulder* is common to many breeds, but when the slope of the shoulder blade is noticeably short and upright, it's not desirable. This upward angle inhibits fluid motion, action, and comfort, and intensifies concussion.

28

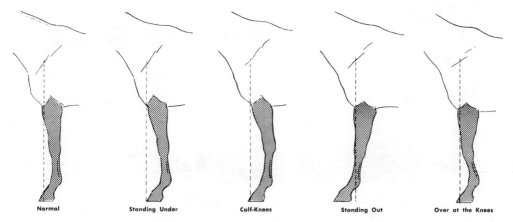

Normal   Standing Under   Calf-Knees   Standing Out   Over at the Knees

Figure 11. The Forelimb—Side View

The upright shoulder occurs because the angle of the shoulder joint is too open, e.g., the meeting of the shoulder blade (scapula) and the humerus occurs at too great an angle. This sets the scapula in an upright position. There's no correction possible.

2. *Standing out* with the front feet places the horse in such a position that he appears to be bracing himself against some invisible pushing force. It stresses the back of the feet, and particularly the tendons and ligaments on the posterior leg surface.

Predisposing problems include navicular disease, joint irritation and injury, and other associated strain injuries and diseases. Forward slanted legs cannot be corrected and should be considered weak conformation.

3. *Standing under* places the feet to the rear of the plumbline and unbalances the horse so it's prone to stumbling and falling. Because the position stresses the entire forelimb, it causes rapid fatigue, lack of sustaining speed, and renders the horse unsafe for pulling, jumping, racing, or gaming.

4. *Over at the knees* makes the horse look as though he's about to kneel down. This deviation is caused by congenital contraction of the flexor muscles at the back of the leg(s), or by racing stress and subsequent injury.

The condition puts stress on the proximal and distal sesamoid bones, both of which act as fulcrums for the flexor tendon. Over at the knees causes joint and bone damage, in addition to injury to the superficial flexor tendon and suspensory ligament.

Since the horse is off balance, he's generally unsafe for speed, running, or jumping events. Matters are seriously complicated if the feet are left too long, since stumbling is a usual consequence.

5. *Calf knees* are the opposite in deviation and are not as dangerous to the rider's safety. Unfortunately, though, calf knees do lead to more

29

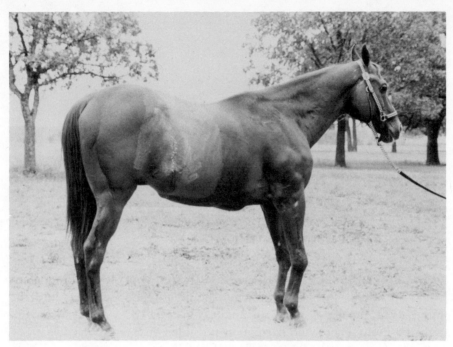

Figure 12. A postsurgical colic case showing severely bucked knees.

damage when the horse is used hard. These problems occur because the unnatural angle of the joint weakens the knee ligaments, irritates and damages the middle knee joint (the joint between the two rows of knee bones), and strains the surrounding joint capsule. Chip fractures of the lower end of the radius and front carpal surface are common, particularly with speed and jumping work.

Due to the abnormal position of the leg, the horse strides by whipping its defective leg down at the completion of each stride, a motion defect known as *pounding*. The concussion produced by this predisposes to damage of the soft and hard tissues of the inner foot.

6. *Upright pasterns*, whether short or long, are not the ideal for any horse. This pastern conformation allows for little flexibility, and so the joints lack proper concussion-coping ability.

If in addition, the hooves are quite small, or equal in circumference at both the coronary band and the ground surface (like a cylinder), the hoof is unable to cope with shock. Upright pasterns predispose to sidebone, cocked ankles, fetlock joint arthritis (traumatic), flexor tendon strain, ringbone, and navicular disease.

7. *Long* and *sloping pasterns* are usually seen on thin, weedy horses with narrow chests and poor development. They're also more prevalent on Thoroughbreds, Saddlebreds, and gaited horses. Such conformation

leads to pedal osteitis, navicular bursae damage, navicular disease, fetlock joint strain, tendon irritation, sesamoid bone fractures, and suspensory ligament damage.

Although long and sloping pasterns give a comfortable ride, they do not hold up well with jumping or running. Slight alteration in the pastern angle is possible with corrective shoeing, but any abrupt or radical change only stresses the pastern area further.

The Hindquarters—Posterior View

The rear of the horse is its driving and power source. To judge the hindquarters for faults, drop your plumbline from the point of each buttock, opposite the tail. Both lines should drop from these points, called the *tuber ischii*, and equally bisect the entire posterior surface of the leg and heel bulbs.

There should be equal distance between the tuber ischii, hocks, and heel bulbs to give the horse a balanced base of support. While most conformation judges advocate this equal distance rule, there's a new one gaining in popularity. This judging standard allows for less distance between the hocks, because many trainers feel the inward deviation gives the horse more drive and agility in jumping and running.

Ideal rear conformation requires enough room between the legs to

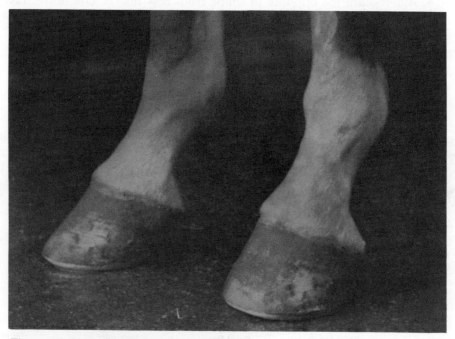

Figure 13. Long, sloping pasterns.

permit good development of the inner gaskin muscles. As with the fore-feet, neither should the rear ones deviate in or out.

Flaws (Fig. 14) found in the hindquarters include:

1. A *wide support base* usually accompanies a lanky body structure and places strain on the inside surface of the hock and leg. The strain is intensified if the horse toes out. Predisposing problems are the same as in the forelegs.

2. A *narrow support base* is common to large, muscled horses, and develops from a twisting of the leg at the stifle or hock joints. It can be accompanied by pigeon-toes. The strain from both defects stresses the lateral surface of the legs, predisposing to the same problems as in the front. Interference is common.

3. *Cow hocks* originate from a hereditary or developmental inner deviation of the points of the hocks, most always seen in a wide support base. The defect is not always common to narrowly conformed horses: stocky ones may also display this fault.

Excessively angled hocks subject the horse to severe medial tendon and ligament strain. This strain, in turn, leads to bog and bone spavin, curb, and irritation of the hock joint and its capsule. Cow hocks are considered weak conformation and are undesirable in extreme cases for breeding prospects, jumpers, or horses asked to do long, hard, or fast work.

4. *Bow legs* are the opposite in shape from cow hocks. The horse has an outward deviation of the bones from the tuber ischii to the hock joints and an inward angling of the cannon bones from the hocks to the fetlock joints.

This out-and-in formation gives the horse a narrow base of support and places a strain on the supportive structures of the legs, especially on the outside aspect of the hock and fetlock joints. In many cases, the

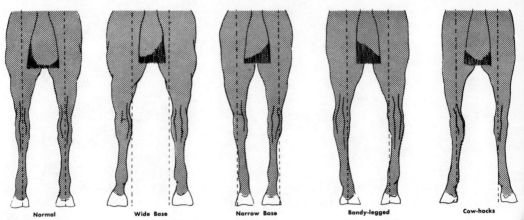

Normal   Wide Base   Narrow Base   Bandy-legged   Cow-hocks

Figure 14. The Hindquarters

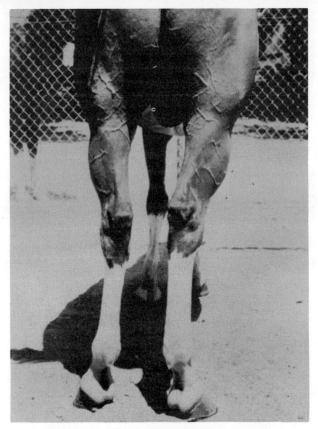

Figure 15. Cow hocks and pigeon-toes.

horse will toe-in, thereby intensifying lateral ligament and tendon strain on the fetlock and pastern.

Since this conformation flaw makes it possible for a straight forward swing of the legs, the horse usually moves with *limber* or *rotating hocks*. Predisposition to hock lameness is greater when this striding defect is present.

5. Strain and injury from *pigeon-toes* and *splay-feet* are the same in the back as in the front.

The Hindquarters—Side View

The ideally built horse should have a fairly horizontal croup with a deep, muscled hip. The stifle and hock joints must be correctly angled to support without stress, and all muscles well-developed and smoothly tapered into the hock area. The cannon, as in the front, should be dense and have firm, well-defined tendons at its back. It's desirable to have the pasterns blend into the hoof at a plane of about fifty to fifty-five degrees some five degrees higher than in the front.

Faults (Fig. 16) of the rear legs, side view, are:

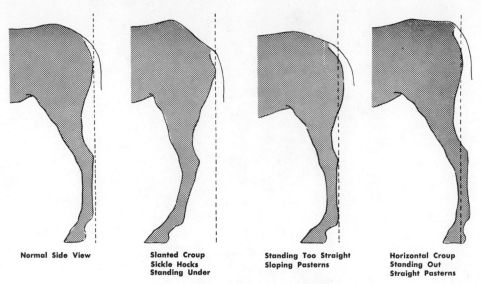

Normal Side View

Slanted Croup
Sickle Hocks
Standing Under

Standing Too Straight
Sloping Pasterns

Horizontal Croup
Standing Out
Straight Pasterns

Figure 16. The Hindquarters—Side View

1. A *slanted croup* is one that drops sharply down from the high point of the hip to the tail base, almost like a dog tucking its tail between its legs. This type of anatomy places the legs under the body and increases strain on the hindquarters. Predisposing problems include joint arthritis, tendon/ligament strain, and curb.

If the defect is slight, many trainers advocate purchase because both the slanted croup and forward deviated legs facilitate getting the legs further under the body. Thus, the horse can jump, stop, pivot, and collect with more ease. You should remember, though, that any deviation of the limbs creates joint stress and misuse of the horse will cause him to develop problems.

2. A very *horizontal croup* sets the rear legs out behind the body. Some breeds have a characteristic straight croup, and should not be faulted for this unless the slant of the croup causes excessive standing out behind. Any excess in this deviation weakens the back and stresses the entire hindquarters.

Collection, handiness, and agility for a horse with a horizontal croup are difficult, and he usually moves with a spraddling motion. The condition is accentuated when accompanied by cow-hocks and turned-out toes.

3. *Standing too straight* behind is caused if the joint angle of the hip or stifle joint is open too far, giving an almost vertical line from hip to foot. When built this way, the horse has no leverage for propelling the body, nor sufficient joint angles to help reduce harmful concussion. In addition, the gaits are stilted and hard on both horse and rider.

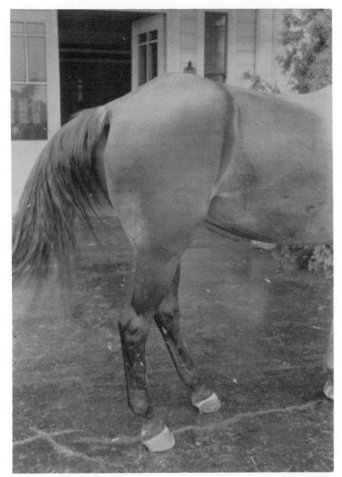

Figure 17. Conformation exhibiting a slanted croup and standing under.

The resulting strain of moving with little or no shock absorption predisposes to an upward fixation of the patella, ligament damage on the anterior surface of the leg, chronic joint capsule inflammation, and chip fractures of the hock (tarsus). If the toes deviate, the strain and effect of any lameness is multiplied.

4. *Sickle hocks* are one of the worse lateral view conformation faults, especially when combined with a steeply slanted croup and cow-hocks. Such a horse has its legs deviating forward from the hock joint; a weak and serious conformation fault. Sickle hocks predispose to ligament stress of the hock joint, spavin, curb, and lateral splint(s).

The Foot—Front and Rear

A good foot is smooth and blemish-free. The soles are concave, thick,

35

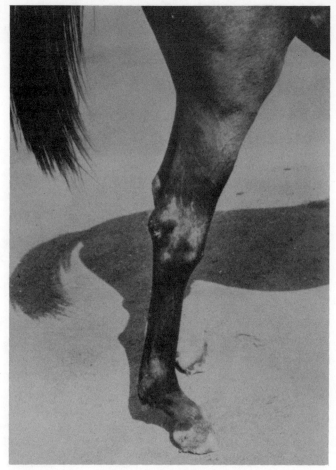

Figure 18. Too straight behind due to tendon weakness.

and the frog large and developed enough to contact ground. The heels are high enough to support the rear of the foot.

Conformation faults in the feet include:

1. *Flat feet* are a hereditary problem that is common to grade horses, heavy breeds, and animals with very wide, round feet. Congenital flat feet should not be confused with dropped soles resulting from disease. This condition can be aided with corrective shoeing.

2. *Mule feet* in horses are so named because of the long and narrow (from quarter to quarter) shape of the hoof. Such constricting conformation is damaging to the internal hoof structures. The tissues within the hoof are unable to contract and relax sufficiently to cope with shock, and predispose to buttress foot (pyramidal disease), ringbone, and sidebone.

3. *Club foot* is a deformity caused by partial contraction of the deep

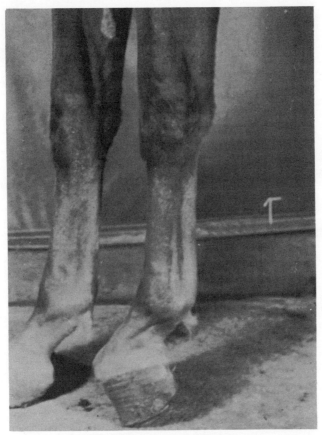

Figure 19. Contraction of the deep flexor tendon.

digital flexor tendon. When the tendon contracts, it causes the coffin joint to remain in a constant, partial state of flexion.

From the side, a severe case appears to be standing on the toe with the very long heel off the ground. One or both feet may be clubbed, and predisposed to pedal osteitis and periosteitis, rotation of the coffin bone, and navicular disease.

The latter problem is caused when the heel is cut down to force the foot into a more normal position. Mild cases often respond to an adequate calcium and phosphorus diet: severe cases in foals to a surgical division of the tendon to restore use of the limb(s).

STRIDING DEFECTS

A horse's *way of going* refers to the direction the legs are carried and how the feet break over to start each stride (Fig. 20). *Breakover* indicates

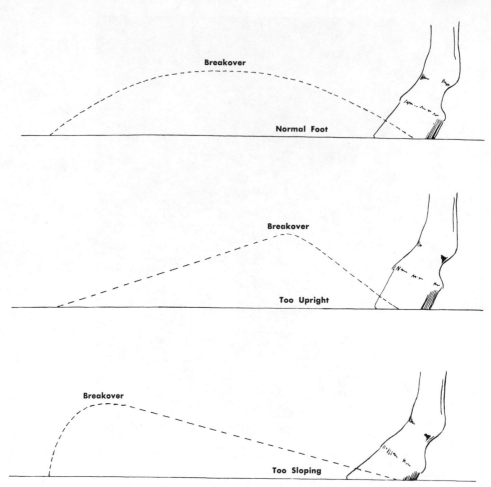

Figure 20. Hoof Angle Determines Flight Path

the point in the beginning of the stride when the heel rises and the foot rolls forward to start its motion. A *stride* is a measure of ground between hoofprints.

Should the horse's heel rise and carry the foot straight forward and over the center of the toe, the direction of the stride will be *true*. If, however, the heel rises and the foot breaks to the inside or outside, it produces a striding defect. The reason for an uneven breakover is a conformation defect, injury, pain, or an unevenly leveled foot. In all cases except pain, corrective shoeing and trimming can correct a *slight* deviation. In more serious cases, protective boots are advocated.

How can you tell if a horse is striding true? Two ways: the first method requires a smooth surface that will hold a hoofprint, and the second, a keen and practiced eye. To test the first method, smooth a

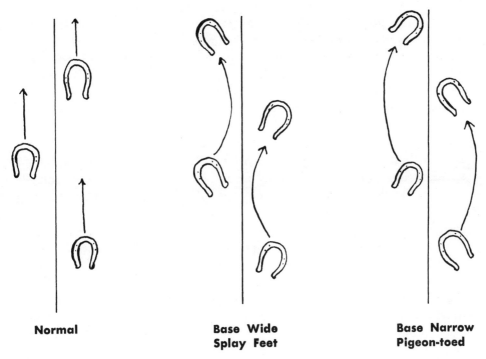

Normal   **Base Wide**   **Base Narrow**
              Splay Feet   **Pigeon-toed**

Figure 21. Tracking patterns.

surface about two hundred feet and draw a straight line down its center. Trot the horse over the line so that the hoofprints appear on either side and parallel to the line. Then look for all prints to point ahead. Any deviation in or out is a clue to a striding problem (Fig. 21).

With the second method, have the horse ridden toward and away from you while you watch the direction of the legs and the breakover pattern of the feet. Often it helps to watch the front legs and feet when the horse is trotted away from you. Then you can line them up with the back legs and give yourself a reference point. The same hint holds true when the horse is coming at you: check the direction of each back leg when the front one is grounded.

Look for the following faults of striding:

1. One of the most common forms of defective striding is when the inside hoof quarter of a leg in flight hits the opposite grounded leg. There are three forms of this fault: brushing, interfering, and knee-knocking.

Brushing is a mild form that is seen as a roughing up of the hair on the inside of the pastern or fetlock. *Interference or striking* is a serious and common form, since it causes bruising, damage to the soft and hard tissue, fractures, splints, and abnormal bone growth. In the forelegs, injury occurs from the knee down, but in the rear, from the fetlock joints down.

Both problems are caused by a base-narrow and splay-footed conformation, cow-hocks, and long, narrow feet. Manmade causes include improper shoeing, fast gaits when tired, overexertion, and riding over uneven ground at fast paces. A good number of young horses, unstabilized in their gaits, stride incorrectly until their joint pain disappears with bone maturity. Protective ankle and splint boots should be used, in addition to having the horse correctly shod.

Knee-knocking is the third form of this striding defect. It's common to narrow-chested horses required to exhibit flashy, hyperflexed gaits at high speed, or until the horse is overly tired. Corrective shoeing offers some relief to the repetitive bruising from one knee hitting the other.

2. *Cross-firing* is a traveling fault generally confined to pacers. In rare cases it may happen to a tired horse moving over rough ground, or in fast going horses with toes deviating in or out. The term refers to striking or hitting the inside of the diagonal forefeet and hindfeet. Bell boots should be used.

3. *Elbow hitting* is mainly seen in gaited or harness horses wearing weighted shoes that are too heavy, or traveling with feet too long. The defect results in the elbow being hit by the heel of the same leg. In severe, or long-standing cases, it can lead to chapped elbow(s).

4. *Forging, overreaching,* and *scalping* are all forms of the same problem—the hindfoot hitting a specific spot on the forefoot of the same side. When forging, the horse hits the hoof or the sole of the front foot with the toe of the hindfoot on the same side. This happens because the forefoot is too slow in breaking over and leaving the ground.

Scalping occurs when the coronary band of the hindfoot hits the toe of the forefoot just as it's breaking over. Overreaching is the most serious of the three, since it involves the heel area and rear surface of the pastern on the front foot.

Overreaching injuries are common to horses in speed and jumping work, since the shoe of the hindfoot can graze or deeply cut the forefoot. Corrective shoeing, plus use of bell boots on the front feet are necessary.

All three problems are common to horses with short backs and long legs, sickle-hocked horses, and those with hindlegs longer than front legs. These faults, in addition, can be complicated or caused by long hooves, uneven trimming, improper shoeing, fatigue, youth, or deep and uneven terrain.

5. *Paddling* and *winging* describe the throwing out of the front feet as they break over to begin a stride. Winging is simply a more noticeable form of paddling seen especially in horses with high knee action. Both forms are caused by pigeon-toes, improperly trimmed feet, and uncollected movement.

Instead of the foot breaking over the center of the toe, it breaks over at the outside. This causes the foot to extend with an outward swing. While there is no direct physical injury caused by this gait to the opposite leg, it does stress both the medial and lateral tendons and ligaments of the in-flight leg.

6. *Pounding* can be seen as well as heard. As the feet are whipped down to complete a stride, they make hard, springless contact with the ground. The accompanying gait is called *rolling*, a sideways movement produced by wide-chested horses with upright, protruding shoulders.

Not only is pounding hard on the joints, tendons, ligaments, and internal hoof parts, it produces one of the most uncomfortable rides imaginable. Horses with straight, upright pasterns are predisposed to this striding defect.

7. *Limber* or *rotating hocks* are prevalent with bowed legs, and predispose to thoroughpin and spavin. The fault is seen from behind as an outward swing of the hock when the foot is grounded.

8. *Stumbling* is a serious problem caused by failure to raise the feet high enough in the strides to clear the ground. Conformation reasons include a narrow chest with poorly formed front legs that weaken with work, standing under in front, improper set of the head and neck (too low), and overly long toes. A horse that is improperly shod, tired, diseased, or injured can also stumble. If corrective shoeing does not alleviate the problem, consult your veterinarian for a physical examination.

9. *Winding, plaiting,* or *rope walking* are all names given to a twisting of the striding front leg around the supporting leg, often with contact. This very distinctive striding fault is common to stout horses with exceptionally wide, muscled fronts.

Such horses generally have a narrow support base and splay-feet, both of which cause the foot to break over to the inside. Interference and stumbling can also occur with severe winding.

2
Equine Psychology and Vices

He flees rather than fight.
He trusts til taught to distrust.
He works willingly until overworked and left without spirit.
He suffers abuse until he learns to fight or find a nervous release.
He communicates with his senses to only a few who will listen.
THIS IS THE HORSE.

To learn equine psychology is to watch the horse react to its environment, companions, and to you. Does he reason with human logic in some situations? In others, does he completely baffle you by his bizzare behavior? Have you ever unraveled a temperament problem by likening the horse's actions to those displayed by a child? If you have, you've gained an insight into equine thinking and reasoning.

The horse is basically a very simple animal with the instinctual ability to problem solve in a very simple manner. Many of his reactions—anger, jealousy, cunning, stubbornness—are universal emotions. Unfortunately, man has complicated these pure survival and pleasure instincts by domesticating the horse and asking him to take on new responsibilities and roles. Thus, the horse's methods of reacting to manmade situations are bizarre, in some cases, and often hard to understand. If you try to do so, by thinking that the horse should react as you would react, you're going to create problems that might have disastrous results for both of you.

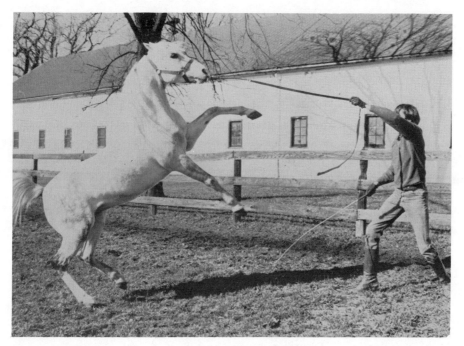

Figure 22. Resistance is a universal emotion for the horse and his trainer.

Reward, punishment, schooling, and management must not be undertaken based on human thinking. A horse does not reason like you, nor does he suffer the remorse and guilt of a dog chastised for a wrong deed. Equine actions following an event, or in response to a demand, follow an elementary *cause and effect pattern*.

Here's a typical example of equine versus human thinking. The horse is being ridden beside a busy road and shies as a truck roars by. What's the typical rider's reaction? Teach the horse not to shy by punishing him with the crop, voice, or legs and hands. Sounds logical according to human methods of punishment, right? But this is a horse: his reasons for reacting, and his understanding of punishment are different.

Let's dissect the event. First of all, the horse acted instinctively and intelligently: he wanted to avoid a potentially dangerous situation, the truck. Fear of the oncoming truck, coupled with the pain from the rider's method of punishment created mental trauma and confusion. Since he was hit for reacting instinctively to what he thought was the right thing to do, the horse will, in the future, associate the truck or car with pain. So the natural reaction will be to shy again because of the expectation of pain.

If the rider doesn't catch on to what's happening, and continues to inflict pain after each shying event, an habitual pattern will be established. Simple cause (motor vehicle = pain) and effect (shying).

What should be done instead of punishing? Most experts advise ignoring the situation, creating a diversion, or soothing the horse when the truck is approaching. When the horse realizes that nothing bad happens to him when a truck or car roars by, he'll gradually ignore passing vehicles.

Many habits are already ingrained and so the area of reschooling rank and spoiled horses is wide open for professional and amateur opinion. If you do need help with a dangerous habit (biting, kicking, rearing), then seek out someone who understands equine psychology and is experienced enough to help you. If, however, you have a horse with few problems, analyze your methods of dealing with him before you react *humanly,* rather, think like a horse.

The equine memory can be an aid or a hindrance in achieving this goal. It directly affects the equine personality, performance skills, and habits. Horses learn by a series of repetitive lessons or happenings. When you begin any phase of schooling in a foal or adult, you must make these lessons as rewarding as possible. If the horse enjoys them, the number of times you'll need to repeat them will be less than if you turn a lesson into a long, boring, or physically painful session.

Don't ever forget that it's not a self-motivated goal for a horse to learn a performance skill or to moderate his natural behavior. He'll do

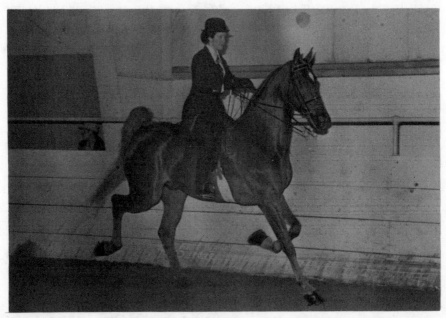

Figure 23. Time spent schooling a horse reaps its rewards in riding a horse responsive to cues and calm in disposition.

it for you because of his willing nature, but his instincts are still on the survival level when stressed.

When you school a horse, it is delightful to have a subject with superior intelligence and the ability to associate response to cue (Fig. 23). Since there are no standard intelligence tests for equines, you'll have to develop a sensitivity to each animal you work with. Treat them all differently, as their temperament demands, and avoid pushing one that is mentally or physically uncoordinated. To ask more of a horse than he is able to give, or to mentally grasp leads to *stress.*

Stress, in turn, eventually manifests itself in discipline problems. If these problems are not dealt with intelligently, correctly, and immediately, they become confirmed habits that may lead to vices.

Not all the blame can be fixed at the point the horse begins his training. In most cases, foals are influenced while still in the womb. Others receive negative strokes from their mothers when they're rejected or orphaned after birth. Rejection by other foals, mishandling during a veterinary examination or foot trimming, or the effects of injury and disease all contribute to a negative mental attitude in the adult.

Stress and Neurosis

Stress is important in creating neurotic tendencies in behavior that can change or alter a horse's personality. Stress develops from a stimulus—fear, confusion, anxiety, pain—that disturbs the horse's normal, balanced state of mind. When that stress becomes too great or is repeated too often, the mind has no other choice than to fight it or avoid it.

When the horse's spirit is strong, he will most often become aggressive in resisting stress: a timid horse generally withdraws and loses spirit. Many horses manage to keep trying to fulfill the rider's demands while diverting their tensions to another source. They exhibit abnormal stall behavior, to be discussed shortly.

What are some of the most common reasons for being stressed? There are as many as there are different personalities of people, standards for punishment, degrees of physical abuse, and types of management. All these factors affect the horse in different degrees, depending on his level of sensitivity.

Some breeds are more susceptible to stress than others because they're high-strung or their jobs are taxing and exciting, as in speed events, open jumping, and racing (Fig. 24). Even within breeds, one horse can take more stress than another, both physically and mentally, without "cracking" under the strain.

This is not unusual: people are the same way. And like people, horses can be overstressed most quickly when they're in poor health or condition, wearing ill-fitting tack or shoes, separated from a companion,

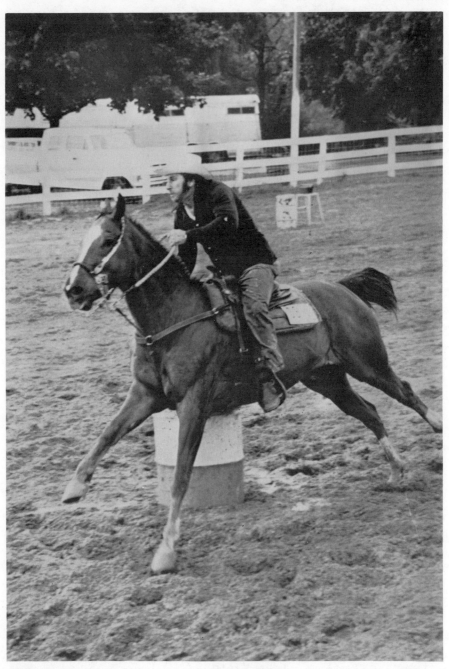

Figure 24. Events such as barrel racing demand a lot, emotionally and physically, from a horse.

or in pain from injury or disease. Physical handicaps also put a tremendous amount of stress on a horse in direct relationship with ability to perform, versus the rider's demand to perform.

Handicaps include poor eyesight and hearing, incapacitating conformation, and substandard motor control. The latter handicap renders the horse incapable of being well-coordinated. He has difficulty with agility, collection, and handling tight maneuvers and jumping courses.

Since most of the stimuli that produce stress and precipitate abnormal behavior patterns are manmade, you can give your horse a better chance of avoiding bad habits by analyzing the following points.

1. Does your horse have performance ability in the area you intend to or are using him? If not, you could be asking too much physically and mentally.

2. Is the horse built well, or are there conformation faults you must take care not to overstress?

3. Are you an experienced rider and trainer, or would you and your horse benefit from professional guidance?

4. Can you tell when you're overworking the horse? Can you quit when the horse is ready but you're not?

5. Are you aware that your schooling routine must be broken up by pasture rest, trail rides, and an occasional vacation from work?

6. Do you know how to read the disposition by watching the ears, eyes, nostrils, tail, and general physical attitude?

7. Are you consistent about giving cues, praise, and punishment? Is your feeding and watering schedule on time daily?

8. Is the horse's health up to its maximum for what you're physically and mentally asking of him?

9. Do you shoe and trim him regularly and correctly? Is the horse on a scheduled worming and immunization program?

10. Do you exercise the horse daily, or at least enough to keep him in condition for what you're asking him to do?

VICES

When a horse shows unpleasant, atypical behavior in response to stress on spoiling (overindulgent treatment), he is said to have a *vice*. This means that the horse's temperament and potential excellence, value, or usefulness are harmed or changed. If the vice is stopped before it becomes an ingrained, permanent habit, the horse is *reclaimed*. When, however, the habit can only be prevented by mechanical means, such as a neck strap for a cribbing horse, the vice is *under control*, but not cured.

There are two categories of vices, *character* and *stall*. Spoiled or rank horses are in the first category and exhibit their abnormal character patterns in two ways: (1) with aggressive behavior toward humans and/or other horses by biting, kicking, striking, crowding against solid objects, and by (2) rebellion against restraint or demands by balking, backing, bucking, rearing, head throwing, prancing, halter breaking, tail wringing, refusal to stand when mounted, and refusal to trailer load, to name a few.

Stall vices are those habits usually caused by nervous tension, and exhibited in the pasture or stall, not against humans or other horses. Stall vices include crib-biting, wind-sucking, wood-chewing, weaving, pacing, circling, pawing and digging, knee-knocking, kicking, tail-rubbing, and bed-eating.

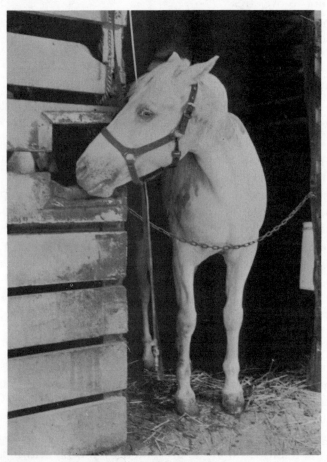

Figure 25. Stall vices, in particular, kicking, can originate because the horse takes a violent dislike to his neighbor.

Before attempting to treat either vice category, have the horse examined for a physical cause. If there isn't one, then ask both veterinary and professional training advice to help you cope with the habit. It's unwise and dangerous for you and the horse to attempt to "cure" a dangerous character vice with amateur opinions or do-it-yourself hints from magazine articles.

With most stall vices, except those which happen in the stall and are aggressive toward you (biting, kicking, etc.), you can attempt treatment yourself. One word of caution—don't employ gimmicks such as hobbles or restraints to effect the cure. Your goal is to try to eliminate or control stress, not add more.

After you check out your horse's physical condition with your veterinarian, you'll have to play detective to find the cause of the vice. Look at your horse's reaction to his stall mates: do they get along (Fig. 25)? Is the horse in a cramped tie stall or a box stall? Are flies irritating him? Is the vice of long standing, or has it just started? Could it have anything to do with recent castration, weaning, heat cycle, recovery from illness, lack of exercise, or change in feeding or schooling routine? Ask and observe, then do it again.

Since most stall vices are caused by tension, boredom, or lack of exercise, what are you doing to perpetuate any of these causes? Why is your horse under pressure? Is your association with him pleasant, or is he frightened of you? Do you ride him too hard or with confusing signals? Are you afraid of him?

When you think you have the answer(s), go to work on it. If you have to use mechanical means to control it, assuming it can't be cured, then you must give the horse a release for his newly developed tensions. Pasture is one of the greatest curatives available to you both. If that's not available, then ride the horse well. Inspect the amount and type of feed you're giving and regulate it according to how much exercise is given. This will often help ease tension caused by excess energy.

Cribbing and Wind-sucking

A horse with the habit of *cribbing* (crib-biting) hooks his top front teeth over any projecting stall part or fence rail, arches the neck, and pulls back to permit air to pass into the stomach (Fig. 27). The air is swallowed by lifting the soft palate in the roof of the mouth.

Because the vice takes so much of the horse's time, the animal often does it instead of, or while eating, and therefore, rarely puts on weight. It also causes excessive wear on the front teeth, may possibly lead to digestive problems, and cause chronic fatigue.

There's no cure, only preventative measures. They include the muzzle, cribbing strap, and an operation, called a myectomy, to remove a portion of the neck muscle. The latter method constitutes a permanent, but dis-

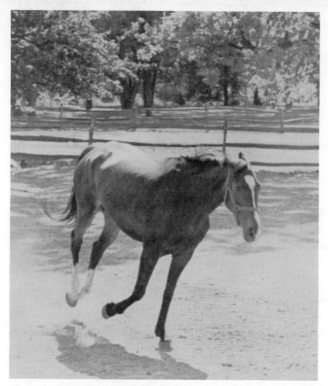

Figure 26. Pasture is a curative for tension.

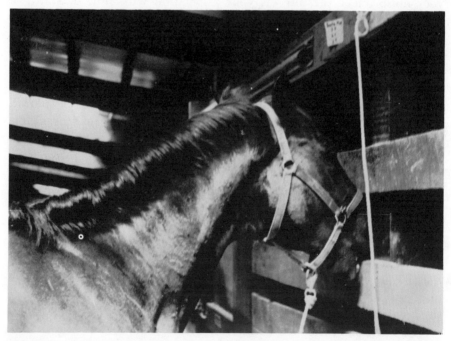

Figure 27. This cribber seized a board to enable him to swallow air and satisfy his vice.

figuring solution to the problem. The muzzle and strap work as long as they're *correctly* placed on the horse.

Don't attempt to prevent cribbing by covering the feed box and stall doors with tires. The horse may chew and swallow the rubber.

The *wind-sucker* "cribs the air," rather than using an object to help him swallow. He does this by jerking his head and neck, and using his tongue to force air into the stomach. Unlike the cribber who can be heard grunting, the wind-sucker may not be immediately detected (beware when buying a horse).

The myectomy is not helpful in preventing this vice, but there is a wind-sucking strap that curtails air-swallowing. Failure to stop the vice leads to loss of flesh, increased flatus, and predisposition to digestive troubles.

Wood-chewing

Wood-chewing, biting, and *licking* are dangerous habits because slivers of wood can become inbedded in the tongue, or lodge in the esophagus and stomach (Fig. 28). These vices can accompany cribbing, and when they do, add to wearing down the teeth. Although blamed on a nutritional and/or salt deficiency, chewing, biting, and licking most often

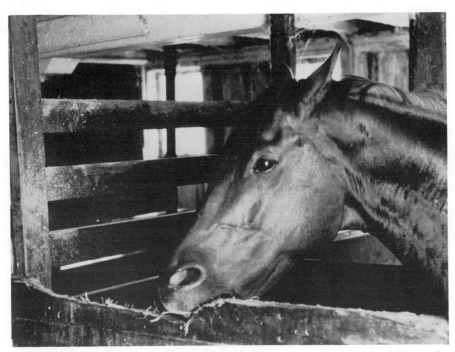

Figure 28. A woodchewer is not only destructive to pasture and stall boards, but he risks damaging himself with splinters.

51

stem from boredom and continue because the horse simply finds them pleasurable.

Preventative measures include muzzling, turning out to pasture, increasing the exercise, and applying a foul-tasting solution to the wooden surfaces under attack. If you use a chemical aid, check first with your veterinarian before applying the solution, since some products contain harmful toxins that may be fatal when ingested in sufficient quantities.

Bed-eating

The most common reason for *bed-eating* is hunger. The habit is also seen in horses given only hay or grass, especially if the quality is so poor the animal suffers a vitamin/mineral deficiency. There is relatively little danger of colic from this vice if the horse is receiving adequate feed and water.

The major harm lies in ingesting chunks of wood, or worm eggs that reinfest the system with internal parasites. To break the cycle while the horse is on worm medication, move him to pasture, change type of bedding, muzzle him, or use a hay net that's removed between feedings.

Tail-rubbing

The most common thought when seeing a horse *rubbing his tail* against a rail or stall side is that he has worms. In approximately one out of ten cases this is true, but in the other nine cases the cause lies elsewhere: scaly dermatitis, dirt in the tail, mange mite infestation, fungus, allergies, or boredom (Fig. 29).

If your horse is on a good, periodic parasitic control program, try treating the problem first with a dandruff or fungicidal shampoo. If this fails, consult with your veterinarian and keep the tail loosely wrapped to prevent hair breakage and raw skin.

In many horses, the habit becomes so ingrained (even after the original cause is eliminated) it should be considered a vice. Turning the horse out more and increasing exercise (two old standbys) will give him less time to stand in the stall and rub.

Knee-knocking

Knee-knocking or *banging* occurs most often when feeding time is near and/or when the horse wants to gain attention from people. It is also common in box-stalled yearlings that are being prepared for sale with good feed and little exercise.

The damage from this habit involves the face of the knee, which is bruised. The injured subcutaneous bursa becomes inflamed and filled with fluid that may have to be drained. If so, the bursa is injected with an anti-inflammatory drug to reduce swelling.

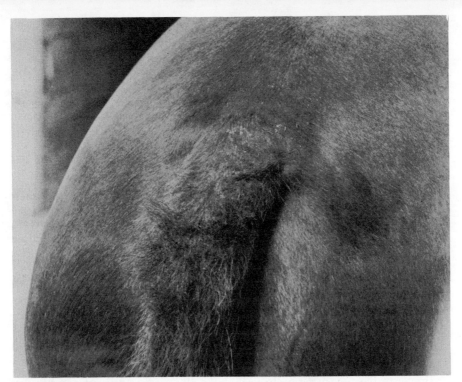

Figure 29. Scaly dermatitis.

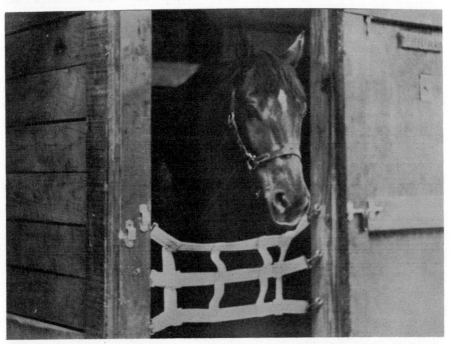

Figure 30. A web gate must be positioned high enough to prevent the horse from putting his feet through the openings and low enough to keep him from crawling out.

To discourage the habit, replace a solid door with a wooden breast bar, rubber-covered chain, or web gate (Fig. 30). You can also try feeding the horse before the others to relieve his anxiety.

Pawing

Pawing often accompanies knee-banging and causes extensive stall damage and a fair amount of wear on the toe of the foot. Tires or hay bales on the floor in front of the stall door (the usual spot to paw), or over the favorite pawing area may curtail pawing. They may also cause the horse to move to a new spot. If so, you can increase the amount of exercise, adjust the feed, or turn the horse out to pasture.

Kicking

Irritability, restiveness, dislike of a neighbor, heat cycle, or sexual excitement in a stallion, and a lack of exercise all contribute to *kicking*. This habit is difficult—if not impossible—to control if you don't have pasture access. A confirmed kicker can strain ligaments and tendons, develop filled legs, capped hocks, sustain cuts and bruises, and possibly fracture the coffin bone.

Preventative measures include kicking chains, padding the stall with old mattresses, or nailing straw-filled burlap bags or tire halves over favorite kicking areas (Figs. 31 and 32). All projecting objects such as mangers and feed troughs should be removed or covered. Protection against capped hocks is important: you may wish to invest in hock boots.

Hobbles, while widely used on kickers, are not recommended for amateur use because they too often lead to casting (the horse goes down in the stall and can't get up) and injury when they are used by an inexperienced person.

Rearing

Rearing in the stall is another vice usually seen in horses that have been kept in too long or are given inadequate exercise. The habit can also result where horses are given excess feed in proportion to exercise, with mares in heat, aroused stallions, playful youngsters, and in angry, abused horses.

If the habit is ingrained and of long standing, be sure the horse is in a stall with a high ceiling. If not, use a leather head bumper. You can also hang water-filled, gallon plastic bottles or tires hung from the ceiling just above head level.

Stall-walking and Circling

The characteristic pattern of pacing to and fro, and circling, continues until a path is worn into dirt floors. Often a contagious vice, *stall-walking*

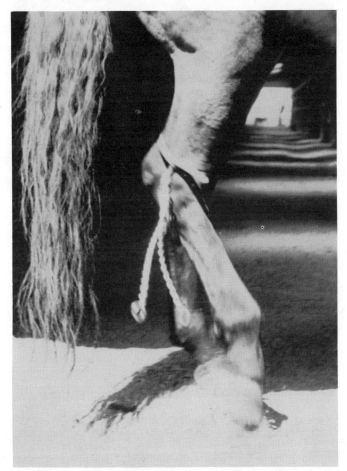

Figure 31. Kicking chains, made from dog collars, deter kicking in many calm-natured horses.

and *circling* are symptoms of hypertension, lack of exercise, boredom, and possible unsoundness.

If you can't exercise or turn out more, cut the feed, especially if your animal is receiving high-protein feed. It's also helpful to give your horse a vacation if he's on an intensive show or training schedule.

Preventative measures include placing hay bales in the movement path, or hanging tires from the ceiling at head level. Don't cross-tie or hobble the horse, since it will increase the stress level and cause injury when the horse struggles to be free. Try to reduce pressure from outside influences before you block his path of motion.

Weaving

Weaving is a side-to-side motion that is almost hypnotic in its rhythm.

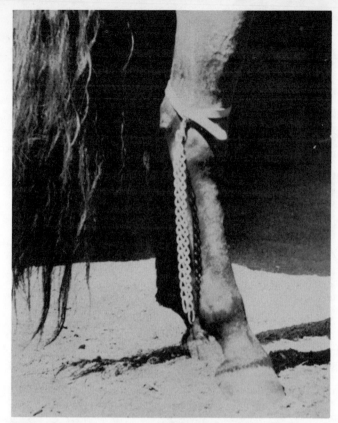

Figure 32. Do not fasten chain tightly around the hock.

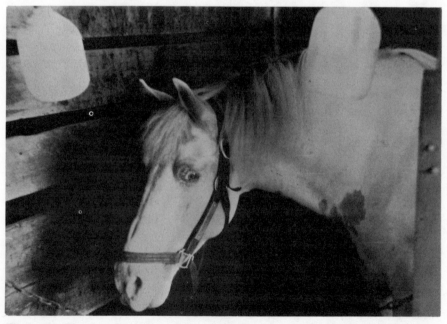

Figure 33. Plastic milk bottles keep this weaver away from his favorite spot.

The causes are the same as for pacing and circling, and the advice for preventing it the same. In long-standing cases, the horse will lose weight, suffer fatigue, and have possible internal foot damage and leg strain. If weaving takes place at the stall door, hang water-filled, plastic bottles on either side of the door (Fig. 33). They'll begin to sway if the horse hits them and, in turn, hit his head as he moves.

3

Let the Buyer Beware

Up to now we've been discussing the horse in bits and pieces, and with objectivity. It's easy to do when presented with a scholastic approach to the inner horse. What happens, though, when the bits and pieces come together in front of you as *the horse* you've always wanted? If you're like most buyers, you lose that objectivity and stand a good chance of buying an unsuitable mount: if, that is, you buy impulsively.

Before you buy—and even before you begin to look—take a lot of time for *prepurchase planning*. You need that time to have a chance to find a horse to suit your present and future riding needs, time and financial limitations, and level of riding experience and patience.

After you've realistically identified these priorities, it's easier to limit the number of available sale horses to the few capable of meeting your needs. Then all you have to do is search for the one with the highest standard of conformation and disposition—no easy task. It's wise to keep one thought in mind: even with the most extensive prepurchase planning, you can still buy a lemon. When you're dealing with living creatures, you can't get an ironclad guarantee of future health or satisfaction.

Finances

Deciding how much to spend is where many people make their first mistake. Too often they set their purchase price too low for the type of horse they want, or try to find a "bargain." As a rule of thumb when

58

arriving at a sensible purchase price, realize that *you usually get quality commensurate with price.* Yes, there are bargains to be found, but usually only for the experienced horseperson who knows anatomy, conformation, and what constitutes a good mover. For the average prospective buyer, such gems are seldom found, even though the seller assures you his horse is a "real bargain."

If you balk at laying out an initial large purchase price, keep in mind that a $150 horse costs as much to maintain correctly as a $1,500 horse. So, set your price realistically for what you want, and buy the best you can afford. Some guides for figuring out cost are:

1. A finished or thoroughly schooled horse will cost more than one with little or no training (a green horse).

2. A *purebred* (horse with registerable bloodlines) is more expensive than a *halfbred* or *grade* (mixed parentage) of the same conformational and mental quality.

3. It's possible to buy a registered, healthy horse from a breeder for a lower price, if that horse does not have show potential or looks.

4. Many breeds, such as the Arabian and Thoroughbred, are so versatile in performance ability, and their breed associations so strong, that they command a higher price for show animals than many other breeds.

5. If you purchase from a professional trainer you pay top dollar.

6. Auctions are a poor place to buy unless the horses are catalogued prior to the sale, and you have a chance to ride and vet them out.

7. An undernourished horse thin from pasture, or an out-of-condition broodmare, will cost less than a sleek, fat horse of comparable quality (Figs. 34 and 35).

8. You generally pay less for a horse being sold in the fall because the summer show season is over, or owners are going away to school, or owners don't want the cost of feeding over idle winter months.

9. Horses over thirteen years of age are usually less expensive than their younger counterparts, unless they are breeding stock with good records or exceptional performers.

Riding Experience

How good a rider are you? Ideally, you should have a minimum of twenty-five lessons from a qualified riding instructor and know elementary grooming, exercise needs, and health requirements. Too often a well-trained show horse is purchased by an inexperienced rider and within two months is ruined because of the timidity and/or abuse of the rider.

There are also many riders—and parents of potential riders—who think a green rider should learn with a green horse. In all but rare cases it

59

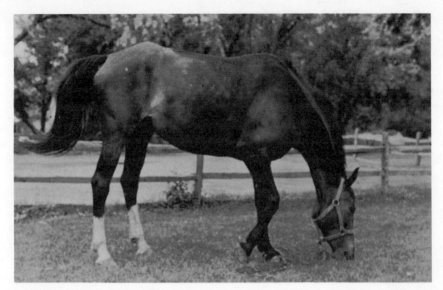

Figure 34 and 35. Two Thoroughbreds: same breeding, different care and management, very different price.

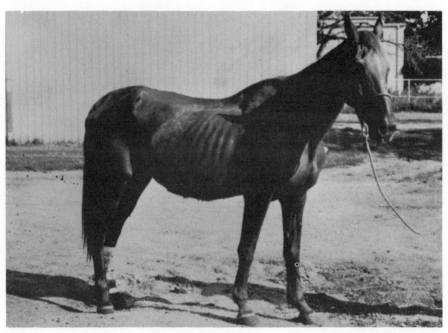

proves to be a disaster. The animal is usually resold as unmanageable, which it probably is after such a confusing and painful experience. Just as a child needs parental guidance and security, a green horse needs the wisdom of an experienced rider. A novice rider also needs the same thing from a well-schooled, older horse (Fig. 36).

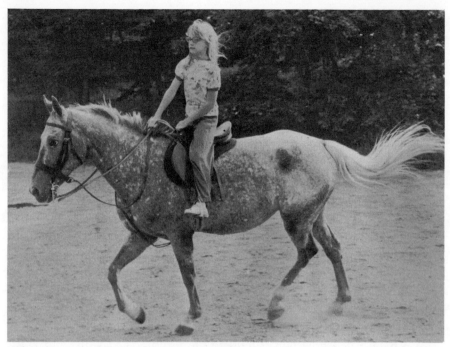

Figure 36. The correct method of finding a suitable mount for a child is to equate the child's inexperience with the horse's experience.

If the future horse owner is a child, his strength, size, and level of riding experience are of prime importance. Children look and feel better on a pony or small horse. If the child is unable to adequately school his mount, the parent should provide an experienced rider to keep the animal in physical and mental condition. Ponies and horses develop dangerous habits when allowed to get their own way.

Available Time

How much time can you spend riding and grooming your future horse? Time is one of the most important considerations in whether you should have a horse. Unless the horse is in pasture, it should be ridden at least five days a week for an hour of moderate exercise. If you're a weekend rider, do you have someone who can exercise the horse for you during the week? Those of you with limited time are often wiser to rent a horse for the hours you have to ride.

Where Is Home?

Is home a pasture, stall, private or public boarding stable, or your backyard? The type of home needed by a horse differs according to his age, sex, temperament, size, level of schooling, breed, and use.

A stallion doesn't go in the same pasture with a mare—unless you're planning a breeding operation—anymore than a high-strung Thoroughbred belongs in a tie stall. If you want your horse in pasture, and it's relatively unwatched, your need will be for a pasture-broke horse that is easy to catch, willing to stay put, and not liable to lose a lot of weight from summer flies and winter cold. Then too, if you have a conformation horse that cannot be blemished, you should look for the closest thing possible to a padded stall.

A good rule to follow is to try and keep the horse in the same or better environment than he was in before.

Purebred or Grade?

After you identify what tasks—performance, pleasure, breeding—your horse must fulfill, you can look further into what breeds or nonbreeds specialize in the same jobs. Is the breed of a horse important as long as the animal can perform the task demanded by you? No, if all you require is a safe, quiet trail horse, or a pony to take the kids for a ride around the yard. Yes, if you want to show or breed the horse you should think about purchasing a purebred.

As a basic rule, show horses tend to be purebreds. If your goal is the show circuit, you'll want to increase your chances of winning by having a horse similar to the ones being pinned in the classes you intend entering.

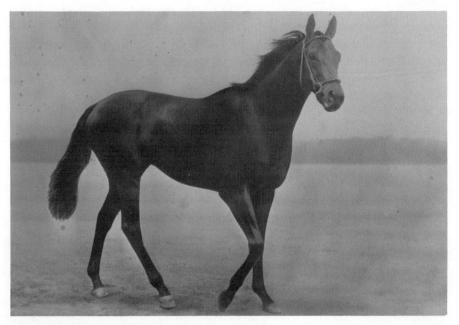

Figure 37. Thoroughbred.

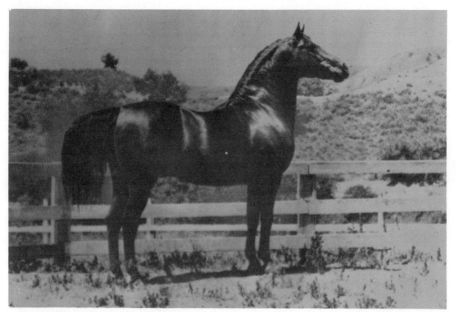

Figure 38. Morgan.

Even though you can enter many classes with a grade horse, few judges will pin you when a recognized breed horse has laid down an equal performance. There are always exceptions in grade-versus-purebred judicial favor, but usually only when the grade is a star performer, and can only be faulted because he isn't registered.

Breeding grade horses is not profitable. The money comes in selling a purebred foal, or in having a registered stallion you can breed to registered mares. Before you purchase breeding stock, consider how much of a demand there is for your chosen breed in the surrounding area. It's often a lot easier and more profitable to sell horses when there's already a demand, rather than having to create your own.

If you decide on a purebred, rather than a grade, next comes the question of what breed to buy. Your choice can often be decided by the job you've intended for the horse. If, for example, you want to show hunters, a trainer will advise you to stick with a Thoroughbred. They usually have the winning edge in flat and equitation classes.

Some breeds are handy doing many jobs. This quality enables you to show the same horse in a stock class and later in a jumping class with an equal chance of winning. Many breed associations, such as Quarterhorse and Paint, to name just two, have breed shows that allow you to participate in many events against your own kind.

One point to remember when trying to select a horse is that each breed has a characteristic conformation that makes it distinguishable

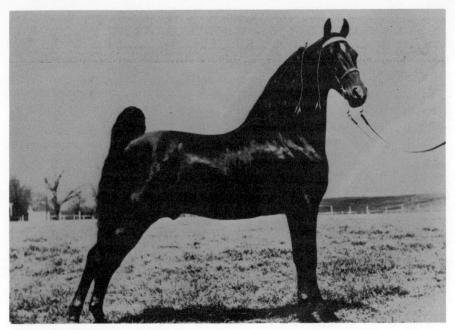

Figure 39. Tennessee Walker.

from others. Within that breed *type* are horses that range from poor to superior in conformation. Some performance tasks demand a certain size, weight, neck length, disposition, or carriage, and this helps narrow down your choice of breeds. Regardless of what breed type you select, you still must look for good conformation above all else. The only breed differences you should take note of are length and slope of back, headset, and length and shape of neck.

Age and Sex

Until five years old, the horse can develop bone and tissue problems by hard riding, long work, jumping, and a heavy rider. Although it would be best to wait until the horse is around four years old to start working him, most are started from eighteen months to twenty-four months of age.

Some veterinarians agree that if the horse is built small and compact, with good bone and muscling, the light exercise given at an early age shouldn't adversely affect bone growth and development. Many more agree that a tall, thin youngster should be trained later, since size doesn't indicate bone maturity. When you buy a young horse, your veterinarian can advise you of joint maturity by taking X rays of the knees and ankles.

Purchasing a foal is an unwise idea unless you already have a horse to ride while the foal is growing, and can take the chance that the foal will not look or perform well as an adult. Even though you buy the product of a sire and dam with good bloodlines and ability, there's no guarantee that their get will turn out with similar talents.

Raising a youngster is a rewarding experience, but if you're looking for a top show horse when full grown, you'd be better off purchasing one now. In the long run, you save money and have the exact horse you want.

An old horse can be as unwise an investment as a very young one. Although many horses that are considered *aged* are only twelve years old, active, sound, and performing well, their resale price tends to be lower than the same caliber horse of lesser years. So if you plan to keep the horse only a few years, plan on buying a young one, as resale will be easier with a preteen horse.

Should you plan on keeping your new purchase forever, an older horse has the advantage of experience and will make a good teacher. It's not uncommon for horses to still be performing well into their twenties.

With breeding stock, the age is not as critical as with performance horses. Mares that are aged can still drop healthy foals, but it's not recommended you buy a maiden mare and try to breed her late in her life. Again, there are exceptions, but veterinarians generally feel a young mare will have an easier first foaling or concepton than an old, maiden mare. Stallions can also breed when well into their twenties. Their ability to transmit genetic characteristics is not affected by age.

The *sex* of your horse is important regardless of the type of riding

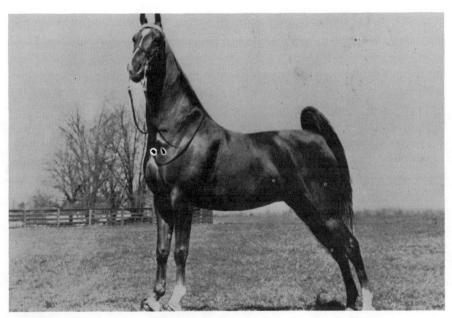

Figure 40. American Saddlebred.

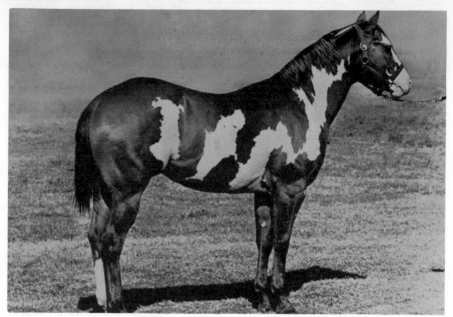

Figure 41. Paint.

you do. Forest preserves, youth classes, and many show classes (group riding) are closed to stallions, but not to mares and geldings. For the inexperienced horseperson, a stallion can prove difficult to manage on the ground and in the saddle.

Mares, too, can be a handful when they come into heat. Many of them, especially when highly bred, are cranky, uncooperative, and hard

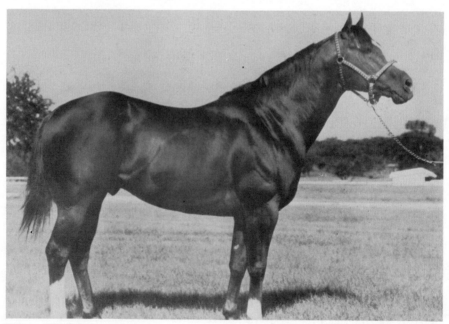

Figure 42. Quarter Horse.

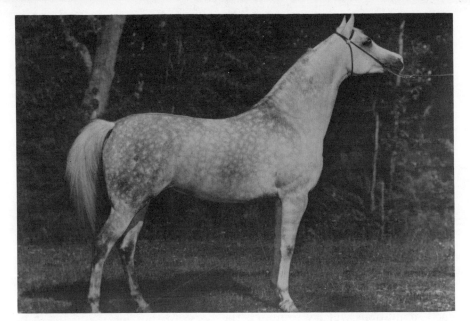

Figure 43. Arabian.

to handle, as they *present* themselves during their cycle. On their nonestrus days, the general tendency is to be a bit more aware of the environmental stimuli than a gelding. Some riders prefer to show a mare, since they feel she puts on a more brilliant performance than a gelding with equal training and ability.

A gelding (castrated male) is usually placid and easygoing. He tends

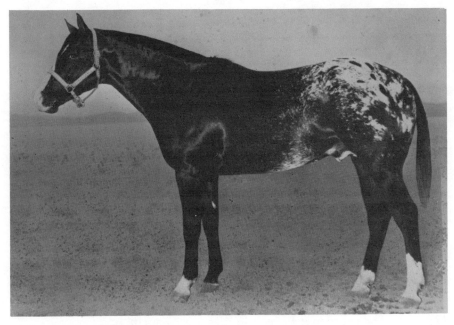

Figure 44. Appaloosa.

67

to overlook more paper, rocks, traffic, and noisy children than a mare.

Remember that these are general observations on sex: every horse is different according to breed, and between horses within the same breed.

Buying Guidelines

You can purchase a horse from many sources—trainers, breeders, private owners that advertise in the paper, friends, or straight out of the show ring—depending on your initial requirements and judging experience.

Buying from a professional is an expensive way to obtain a horse if you're worried about money. It does, though, have advantages. A trainer has access to a lot of horses and can generally come up with what you want: his searching time is calculated in the purchase price. You're also paying for his professional opinion on whether the horse is a good mover, tidy jumper, ready for the ring, and right for you. Trainers with good reputations will try to match the horse to the rider—and make a profit—because continued business depends on having happy customers.

With most professional dealers, you also have the option of a pre-purchase trial period, or a return guarantee, meaning the horse may be

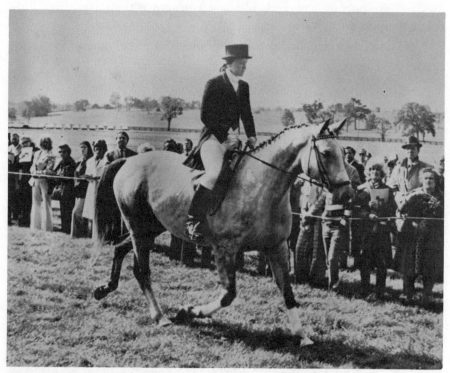

Figure 45. Trakehner breed excels in dressage competition.

exchanged for something more suitable within a certain time period.

Purchasing a horse from an ad can be risky. Haven't you asked yourself why such a fantastic-sounding horse is being sold for such a low price, or why an owner worded the ad "$500 or offer"? If you know what you're looking for and are sure about the elements of good conformation and soundness, or can take an experienced person along, then try looking at ad horses.

You'll usually pay less here than through a dealer, but you'll probably have to forego the prepurchase trial or return guarantee. Because of this, take care to have a prepurchase examination and ride the horse as much as you can before signing a check.

The method of buying from the show ring is mainly done by people willing to pay top dollar for top performance. Its advantage is that the buyer can see the horse in action and view performance skills in competition (Fig. 45). Since many show horses are tranquilized or given pain killers before the show, their performance is not always a true indication of their soundness.

Regardless of the method you use to find a horse, heed the old adage, "*let the buyer beware.*" When you're considering a horse for purchase, check the following points:

1. Take along an experienced person or a veterinarian.

2. View the horse first in its stall to see if it has stall vices. Look at the wooden partitions to note chewed wood, and then at the side walls for indication of hoof marks from kicking. Also note how the horse greets you—friendly, curious, annoyed, distant, disinterested.

3. Watch its reaction to being tacked up and look at the type of bit and equipment used.

4. If the horse is too young to be ridden, have it longed. If ridable, ask the seller to mount first and watch how it stands (or doesn't) when mounted, accepts cues, moves out, and if it appears lame. Jumping form and performance skills should be analyzed by an expert in those fields if you're not sure what you're seeing.

5. After the horse is worked for you, try him yourself.

6. Note whether the breathing is labored or the walk and trot are unsound.

7. Visit the horse—unannounced to the seller—several times before you commit yourself.

8. Ask the seller to trailer-load the horse and also see how it hauls.

9. Does the horse object to clipping, grooming, braiding, picking out the feet, etc.? Ask how it acts when ministered to by the veterinarian or shoer.

10. What type of shoes are worn and where are they worn out?

11. Color shouldn't be important unless you're going to breed for

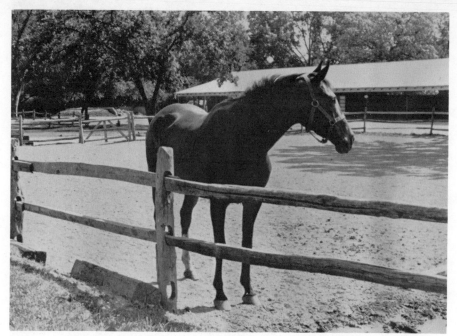

Figure 46. Observe the horse at pasture—is he calm and easy to catch?

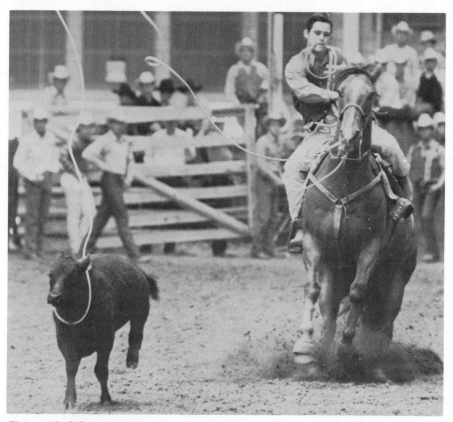

Figure 47. When purchasing a finished horse for a specific task, be sure to watch him work before you buy.

color or are showing in classes that frown on anything other than the standard black, bay, or grey.

12. If the horse will be out in pasture should you buy him, ask what he's like in pasture and turn him out to see for yourself. Does he remain calm and content to stay there, or does he jump out or push on the gate?

13. Will the owner allow a prepurchase examination? If not, move on to another horse.

14. When you buy a mare in foal, or a mare for breeding, find out about her foaling and breeding habits. Obtain a certificate from your veterinarian that the mare is in foal and/or has healthy reproductive organs free of disease.

15. Use a veterinarian of your choice for the exam. When it's over, obtain a statement that the horse was checked and have any problems or blemishes noted. Also have the seller sign a statement saying that the horse is free of riding and stall vices, to the best of his knowledge.

If you're working with a professional dealer, get an agreement that if the horse doesn't work out within a specified time limit, you can return or exchange the horse.

16. Get the horse's medical history, shoeing problems, mental quirks, and feeding schedule before taking him home.

Unsoundness

The terms *sound, serviceably sound, unsound,* and *sound at halter* refer to the absence or presence of disease, injury, and conformation flaws that affect the serviceability of the horse. A *sound* horse is one that cannot be faulted in any physical way, from the inside out.

Serviceably sound means the horse has some problems structurally, but is sound for the purpose that you intend for the horse, be it breeding, pleasure, or show. The term *unsound* means the horse has something wrong that will affect his ability to perform in the expected manner of the purchaser. Some veterinarians prefer to use *sound at halter*, implying only that the horse can stand and wear a halter, nothing else.

Unsoundnesses include:
blindness and other eye problems (some correctible)
bone and bog spavins
bow tendons
conformation defects that predispose to unsoundness
congenital mouth defects (undershot jaw and parrot mouth)
cryptorchid, monorchid
curb
dental diseases (some correctible)
founder

heaves
hernia
hoof diseases (thrush, corn, sandcracks, gravel, quittor)
infectious diseases
navicular disease
reproductive tract diseases or abnormalities
ringbone
roaring
sidebones
splints
stringhalt
sweeny
tumors

Blemishes

Blemishes are external scars, sores, firing patterns, hairless spots, split or torn ears and/or nostrils, bite wounds, tail defects, and calcium buildups that mar the looks, but not the performance. Additional blemishes include windpuffs, bursitis, hygromas (Fig. 48) or swellings. shoe boils, and capped hocks and elbows.

While these marks do not affect serviceability, they do lose halter points and often cause disqualification in conformation classes. Blemishes

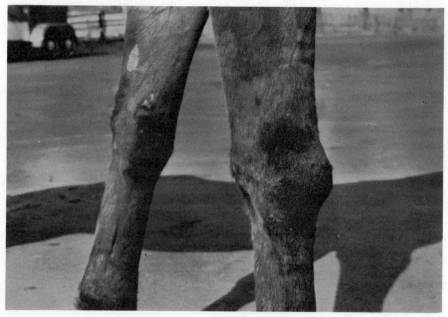

Figure 48. Hygroma, or swelling, on the right knee.

that result from the performance of the horse's job, as in hunter classes, are not counted for disqualification.

Vices

Vices, as discussed in the preceding chapter, can present a deterrent to purchase just as blemishes and unsoundness do. While many vices can be dealt with or prevented, a great number are physically harmful and place a hardship on the owner. It's the seller's obligation to make you aware of a confirmed vice before the sale so that you may consult a trainer or veterinarian as to the seriousness of the vice.

Insurance

If you own a horse costing in excess of $500, you should consider *insurance*. It's an important financial consideration that's almost mandatory when the horse is an expensive show or breeding animal. Many agencies deal exclusively with equine insurance and are familiar with the performance requirements of different show and class events. They offer policies to cover death by (1) fire, lightning, and transportation, with coverage limited only to these three causes, (2) accidents, which includes the preceding policy coverage, plus any outward accidental causes of death, and (3) full mortality, which includes death from any cause including the first two, plus diseases, illness, etc.

You can also buy, for additional cost, specialized coverages such as loss of use, unborn foal coverage, theft, trip transit, and stallion infertility. With the loss-of-use policy, the insurance company will pay a percentage close to the insured value of the animal if the horse is injured so he cannot be used for the purposes for which he was orginally insured. The animal may not be seriously injured, but is rendered useless for his specified job.

The unborn foal coverage insures the foal from the time of breeding to a specified period after birth, usually until the foal stands and nurses. The mare in foal is required to be swab tested before her first service of the season, have normal genital organs, be manually examined at forty-two and forty-five days for presence of twins, and be confirmed of pregnancy by a manual and/or blood test. Her health must be excellent, with all cases of colic reported, vaccinations noted, and former foaling history given.

Stallion infertility covers the value of the stallion in the event he is unable to breed. Theft coverage is self-explanatory, and trip transit covers death of the horse during a specified period of shipment by land, air, or sea within the United States or foreign countries.

An insurance examination can be given at the time of the prepurchase vet out and mailed in up to ten days after the exam. If the horse's coverage is being raised after a period of time, the animal will have to be re-examined. Any of the above policies can be taken out on your breeding animals if they are leased by another person for use over a specified length of time.

The majority of insurance companies will not accept for insurance purposes those animals which exhibit vicious tendencies, those suffering recurrent attacks of colic or bleeding, tubercular horses, or those which have been denerved for navicular disease. A horse that has been fired or blistered may also be uninsurable if there is any likelihood of future danger to life or limb as the result of such procedures.

4

General Management

General management is the area of horse care that includes the handling, exercise and stabling requirements, and daily ration needs of your horse. It's an important part of maintaining health and service-ability, even though it may seem cut-and-dried at times. A horse, when properly managed on the ground and under tack, is less likely to succumb to diseases and injuries that befall the neglected and misused animal.

Restraint

If your horse is hard to hold for clipping, shoeing, or veterinary examinations, you can utilize several *restraint methods* to accomplish your goal with little or no trauma to either of you. Start with patience, firmness, and an understanding of why the horse is reacting negatively. Is he frightened because he's never experienced what you plan to do to him? Has he had a bad experience before and anticipates pain? Is he simply a rank individual who will fight anything? Sizing up the situation will afford you the best method of restraining the horse with the least amount of trouble.

Choose a restraint commensurate with the personality of the horse and the amount of handling and training he's had. This means a little for a trained and reliable horse, more with a gentle, but green or young horse, and a lot for a spoiled animal. Whichever method you choose, it shouldn't create more fear and pain, or make the horse's disposition worse.

The *lead shank* with a chain is effective on young and/or nervous horses when you lightly tug on it or shake it to gain their attention. You can also use it to pull the head to one side to avert biting or pawing. For more control, pass the chain over the nose. Many professionals pass the chain under the chin, through the mouth, or over the gums to check behavior. If your horse is not used to these methods, it's best to avoid them. Too much pressure on the chain will cut the skin and create enough pain that the horse will learn to fear the sight of the chain.

The *twitch* works by putting pressure and pain on the upper lip. It can be a rope or chain loop through a wooden handle, or a do-it-yourself twitch that clamps on and needs no attendant to handle it. The most effective way to use a handle twitch is to slightly twist the handle to alternate lip pressure. This avoids deadening sensation in the lip. At no

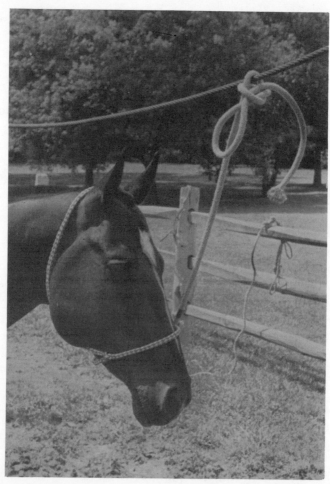

Figure 49. A slip-knot and an overhead rope make a good safety combination.

76

time use a twitch on the ear, since the cartilage and nerve can be damaged.

Lifting the tail gently over the back works on foals, ponies, and horses. When you use this method on a small animal, put one arm around the chest and use the other to hold the tail. On large animals, have someone hold the head rather than tying up the horse. Caution should be used when lifting the tail, since too vigorous handling can injure the tail.

Holding up a leg works well for kickers. If the horse is being shod, for example, in the left rear, then lift the front right—and so on—to dissuade kicking. If you're working alone, do not strap or tie up the leg, since the horse can easily go down when struggling to free himself.

Tying the horse is effective if your equipment is strong and the horse is not left alone in this position. Use a strong halter (preferably nylon), a thick rope tied above shoulder height with about two feet of slack in the rope, a quick release knot, and a pole that won't break or loosen (Fig. 49).

GROOMING

Daily grooming is essential for a stall-boarded or sick horse regardless of whether you work the animal. Brushing stimulates circulation and

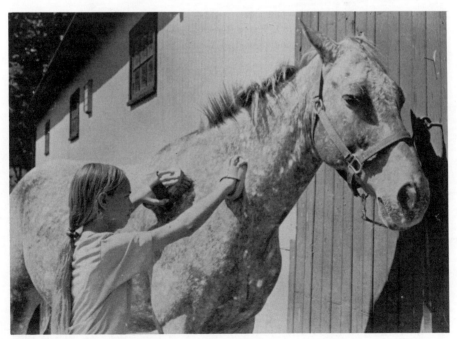

Figure 50. Currying a horse is a daily, essential part of good management.

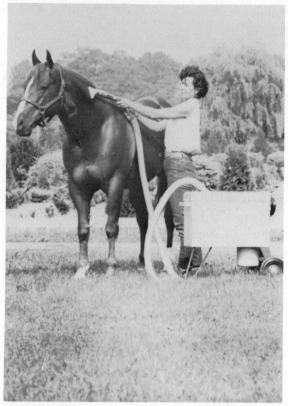

Figure 51. Vacuum grooming a horse is easier on you than brushing and also stimulates and deep-cleans the skin and coat.

tones muscles, removes dirt and sweat, and keeps the body relatively free of parasites. It also gives you a chance to inspect the horse for cuts, swellings, and soreness.

Equipment need not be elaborate or expensive. Buy a stiff body brush, soft finishing brush, face brush, and a plastic, oval curry. You'll also need a hoofpick, sweat scraper, mane comb, and several cloths and sponges.

Groom the horse before and after you ride—about a twenty-minute job if you do it thoroughly. Start with the mane and tail. To eliminate snags and problems with burrs, you can spray on a coat conditioner that leaves the hair silky and tangle-free.

Next take the curry in one hand and the body brush in the other. Use the curry in small circular patterns to raise dust and loose hair and wisk it down and out with the brush. Every few strokes, pass the brush over the curry to remove hair and dirt. When you get to the legs, use only the brush. Polish off the horse with the finishing brush and a cloth.

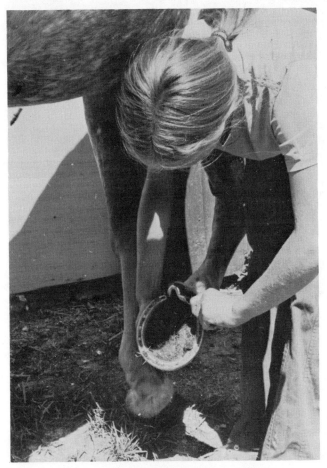

Figure 52. Pick the feet before and after each ride to remove stones and check for bruises of puncture wounds. Don't neglect picking the feet of a stall-bound horse, since thrush loves an untended foot.

Before you groom after a ride, have the horse cool and dry by walking for about fifteen minutes. If there's mud on the legs, wash it off with warm water or wait until it dries to brush it off. Never leave mud on the legs, since skin irritations can develop (Fig. 53).

The feet should be picked out by taking the hoofpick and working it down the V-shaped frog grooves toward the toe. Look for stones that have lodged between the sole and the shoe, and for objects that might have penetrated any part of the foot. When riding out in wet weather, apply a film of Vaseline over the heel bulbs and backs of the pasterns to protect them against drying and irritation. Once a week use a commercial hoof dressing to keep the hoof moist and retard cracking.

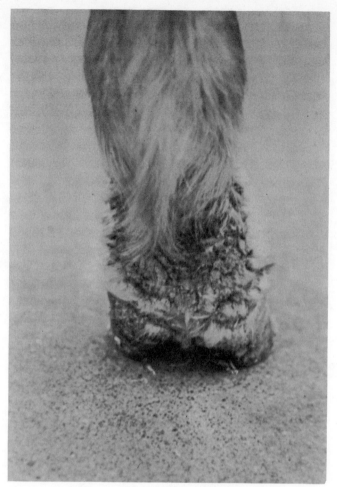

Figure 53. Extensive skin cracking and scabbing at the rear of the pastern.

Bathing

A *bath* is no substitute for good grooming with a brush and curry: use them together to keep the coat clean and shiny. During cold-weather months, and when there's a chance that the horse cannot be thoroughly dried before you put him away, don't bathe. There's a risk of chill.

Regardless of the outside temperature, avoid using cold water directly from the tap. The ideal water temperature is temperate. If you can't hook your hose to a hot and cold faucet system, use buckets of warm, soapy water with one part lanolized soap to three parts water. When you're done, rinse well to remove soap residue from the skin. Remove excess water with the sweat scraper.

Many owners squirt water from the hose directly into the horse's face and then get mad when the horse backs away. Horses dislike water in the face, especially when it gets into the ears (Fig. 54). So use a cloth or sponge on the head. Don't use the sweat scraper on the face or other bony areas.

The last step to bathing is to walk the horse til dry or put him out to graze in the sun, if the weather is hot.

Care of the Genitals

The *mare's bag*, located between her rear legs, should be washed weekly, since dirt and body waste accumulate in a deep groove between the teats. This causes an itchy buildup that looks like black flakes when removed. Gently work on the area with warm water and a soft cloth until all dirt is gone: finish the job with a thin film of baby oil to keep the skin soft.

The *male's penis* also needs attention to remove flaky dirt and body wastes accumulating in the space between the penis and its surrounding sheath. In addition to keeping this area clean, there's a small pouch directly above the urethral opening of the penis that collects waste material (smegma). When it hardens, a "bean" is formed that can cause constriction of the urethral opening.

Have your veterinarian attend to this once a year. He will usually tranquilize the horse to stimulate a relaxation and dropping of the

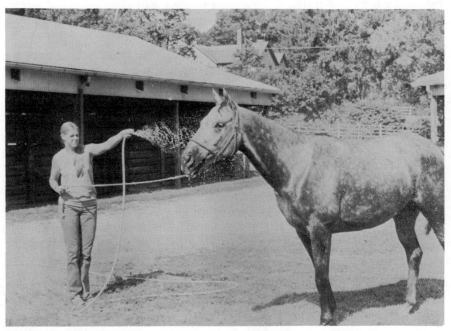

Figure 54. Few horses enjoy water in the face as much as this polo pony.

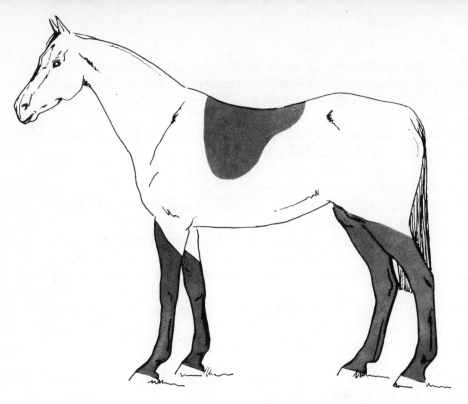

Figures 55 and 56. These clipping patterns are applicable to both English and Western-ridden horses that are used outside during cold months. Hair is left on the legs to afford extra protection, since there is no fat to insulate them. The belly and throat are trimmed to allow fast evaporation of sweat. If the weather in your area is extremely cold, Figure 56 is an ideal pattern to provide protection, while permitting cooling to take place.

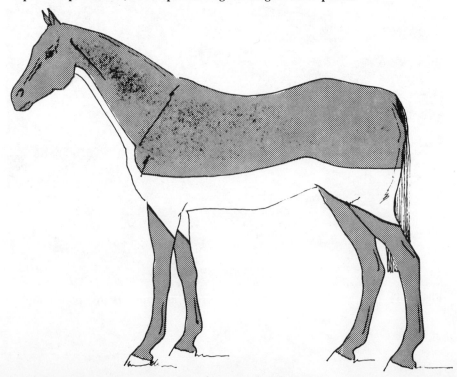

penis before cleaning him with soap and water. Don't attempt this yourself until you see how your horse reacts to the process. Many animals kick, not because it's painful, but because it's uncomfortable or strange to them. If you own a breeding stallion, his penis should be cleaned before and after each service.

Clipping

The sound of *clippers* panics most uninitiated horses, and tranquilizing may be the only way to quiet the horse for clipping. Other horses will quiet if they're introduced slowly to the sound and feel of the clipper vibration.

Once you can get next to your horse with the clippers turned on, stroke him with the clippers held in your hand so he can feel the vibration through your fingers. If still calm, begin clipping against the grain of the hair, rear to front, and make each cut as long as possible to avoid a patchy job.

Horses stabled indoors during the winter do not usually develop a heavy coat if blanketed from the first onset of cool weather. If you ride in an indoor ring over winter months, clipping in the fall and blanketing are advised. This procedure permits quick evaporation of sweat, and avoids a long cooling period. For the horse that alternates between indoor and outdoor riding, clip the body only and leave the hair on the stomach and legs. It may not look as tidy as a complete clip job, but it will help avoid chilling during cold rides.

Mane and Tail Care

Depending on what breed you own and what riding style you prefer, the *mane* can be roached (clipped off), pulled short, or left long and natural.

When you thin and shorten the mane, take about ten hairs in one hand and the mane comb in the other and backcomb the hairs. When you have about five hairs left, wrap them around the comb and yank down. Start with the underneath hair and avoid jerking out too many at a time or the skin will become sore.

If the mane won't lie down flat, use a gel hair setting preparation, a neck hood, braids, or weights to train it to the proper side. Don't leave braids in too long or the hair will break and give a ragged appearance.

Before you attempt to thin out the *tail* or shorten it, ask a professional trainer to advise you on the process and the correct length for your horse's conformation and way of going. When the tail is thinned, you can avoid breaking hairs by combing the tail with your fingers, rather than a brush or comb.

Blanketing

A *blanket* can be used to keep the coat clean, coat hairs light, absorb moisture from the coat when the horse is walked after exercise, and to raise the temperature of a sick horse. Blankets are available in different weights and weaves for all temperatures and weather conditions, rain to snow.

Don't blanket a horse left in pasture or leave a blanketed horse out in the rain unless its cover is waterproofed. In the stall, use a surcingle or roller to keep the blanket in place so it doesn't became entangled in the horse's legs. When you adjust the web straps on the blanket, cross them under the belly and leave enough slack for the horse's ribs to fill out when he lies down.

FITTING TACK

Tack, or gear, refers to pieces of equipment used on the head and body of the horse as an aid to the rider's safety, as a communication device, to facilitate a specific job, to control the horse, and to aid in its training. Each piece must be fitted for the comfort of the horse and used with gentleness and knowledge to secure the best results.

There are two basic bit types—the *snaffle* and the *curb* (Fig. 57 and 58). The snaffle bit induces flexion by putting pressure on the tongue and corners of the lips. It works like a hinge on the tongue, and has a tendency to raise the head. The curb lowers the head and achieves flexion of the poll and jaw by putting pressure on the poll and the chin groove.

With a snaffle bit, the fatter the mouthpieces and the tighter the

ENGLISH RIDING BITS

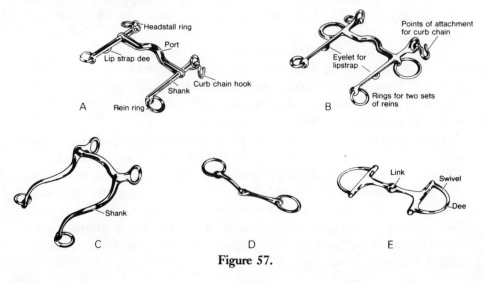

Figure 57.

84

WESTERN RIDING BITS

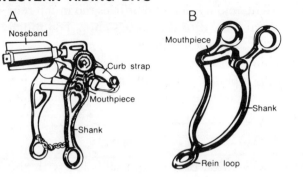
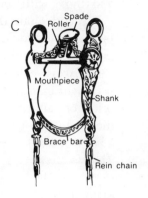

Figure 58.

joint between them, the more gentle the bit's action. A harsh snaffle has straighter, narrower, and more pointed bars with a loose joint between them. A curb bit increases in severity with the length of the shanks and the height of the port, plus type (chain versus strap) and tightness of the curb strap.

The curb operates on the principle that, as the reins are pulled back, the headstall lowers as much as one inch for every two inches of backward rein pull. Long cheek pieces on the bit may be in vogue with some riders, but usually cause the horse to carry its head at an improper, unbalanced angle and allow the bit to fall forward to an uncomfortable position in the mouth.

When the snaffle is combined with the curb bit in a bridle, it is called a *full bridle* or *Weymouth*. Each bit is used both independently and together to control and position the head. It's considered an effective schooling bit for both English- and Western-ridden horses.

When you fit a bridle and bit, there are quite a few points to remember to achieve control and make the horse comfortable in his tack.

1. The width of the bit must fit the width of the horse's mouth. If too narrow, it will pinch: if too wide, it will not work effectively and will be uncomfortable in the mouth.

2. When the cheekpieces of the bridle are properly adjusted, there should be one definite wrinkle at the corner of the mouth. If the bit is too low in the mouth, there is no wrinkle: too high and there are too many wrinkles and too much pressure.

3. A dropped noseband is used with a snaffle bit to keep the horse's mouth closed and give better control. It should never be used with a curb bit, since the action of the combination is too severe.

4. The use of a martingale to keep the horse's head down increases the severity of a bit, since the animal cannot evade the bit's action when it becomes painful. This is particularly true with standing martingales

and those with wire nosepieces, as opposed to running martingales.

5. A curb chain that is too tight, and a rider who utilizes too much rein pull combine to form a potential hazard to the horse's chin. Too much pressure can bruise or break the underlying bones.

6. Excessive fretting with the bit, head-shaking, or change in temperament can be caused by poor hands, ear problems, or an ill-fitting bridle or painful bit. In some cases, teeth problems can be irritated when the bit moves against the teeth.

The Hackamore

Western horses are more likely to be broken and schooled with the rawhide *bosal* or the *mechanical hackamore* than English-ridden horses. Both are substitutes for the bit—whether temporary or permanent—and are very effective for green horses and those with a damaged mouth.

The bosal is a teardrop-shaped rawhide piece that attaches to a headstall and has reins tied to the heel knot at the base of the bosal. Its severity depends on the size—the thinner, the more severe—and the stiffness of the rawhide. The length and width also vary according to the anatomy of the horse's head and the leverage needed to control the horse and set the head. The bosal puts pressure on the nose and lower jawbones, both of which can be severely damaged with too much pressure.

The mechanical hackamore has a noseband of leather or covered wire cable, a chin strap or chain, and long metal shanks that apply pressure on the nose and poll with rein pull. It is used without a bit, like the bosal, and fastens onto a headstall.

One of the most undesirable features of using the bosal or machanical hackamore is erroneously positioning both too low on the nose. This constricts the air passages, is painful, and may cause the horse to fret or rear when pressure is applied. A correctly fitting nosepiece sits above the cartilage area on the front of the face, resting on the bony bridge of the skull (Fig. 59).

The Saddle

When you fit a *saddle* to your horse, check the height of the withers, width of the back, and breadth of the shoulders. The saddle tree should be wide enough to avoid pinching a broad horse and narrow enough not to lie flat on the spine of a thin horse. The pommel is an important feature with prominent withered horses. It can be a source of irritation and bruising if it rubs the withers. A cut-back saddle will eliminate this problem as will a pommel pad placed between the withers and the saddle.

When you put on the saddle and pad, position the saddle close to the

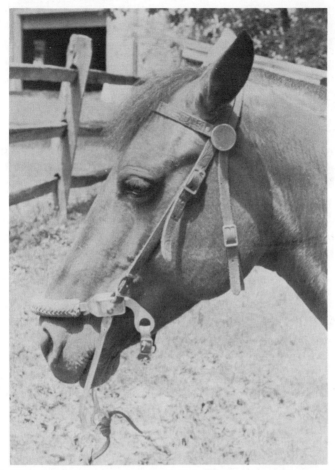

Figure 59. This mechanical hackamore is too large for the horse's head and placed too low on the nose. Note that the curb chain is not properly positioned in the chin groove and will cause jaw bone damage the way it is set.

withers and rock it gently until it settles into the small of the back. Before you tighten the girth or cinch, take up a longitudinal fold in the pad or blanket to form a channellike air space under the length of the saddle. This precaution will keep the blanket or pad from tightening over the back and withers and allow some air to circulate over the back.

After riding for a while, your pad may bunch up under the saddle skirts. Instead of yanking it forward, dismount, lift the saddle, and reposition the blanket. The object is to keep all the hairs flat and avoid irritation from hairs pulled forward with the blanket.

For those of you who ride for hours on end, allow a few minutes per hour to lift the saddle and freshen the back. Keeping the saddle off the pressure areas along both sides of the spine permits blood to recirculate through those areas. These spots go "dead" after a time, thus leading to saddle sores and possibly a cold back.

If your horse is bothered by *saddle sores*, you can cut holes, over the sore spots, in a felt saddle pad. Should sores develop while you're on a trip away from home, begin applying cold packs for twenty to thirty minutes to reduce swelling and relieve pain. Cortisone cream rubbed into the sore area will reduce swelling and induce healing. When you tack up again, reposition the saddle blanket and remove all wrinkles.

Treatment for *cinch sores* on a trip is the same. Using a leather or sheep-wood protector over the cinch rings will guard against tenderness in the area. These sores heal most quickly with rest.

The main object in healing is to keep the sores moist, so a scab won't form. Scabs tear off and increase irritation and danger of infection. Air the back frequently, keep cream on the sores, and stay still in the saddle when you ride.

Tack Care

Leather is preserved and kept pliable by removing dirt and sweat and by renewing the lost animal oils with a periodic application of commercially prepared lanolized oil. Glycerine soap oils and cleans, but it's sticky and needs to be wiped well after each application. Saddle soap—without a softening agent—produces a hard polish and shine because of the beeswax in it. Alternate between these two when you clean and occasionally use a leather preservative to give long life to leather.

Tack should be cleaned after each use with a damp sponge. If you allow dirt and hair to accumulate and cake, the rubbing of the dirty leather against the horse's skin will usually cause sores. When you don't use a saddle pad, you'll need to clean the saddle more frequently with soap. The same hygienic attention you pay to leather holds for cleaning the pad or blanket.

Neither tack nor grooming equipment should be used for more than one horse unless it's cleaned and disinfected to prevent the spread of skin diseases. You can buy a fungicidal disinfectant at a tack store to wipe your tack and soak brushes and combs. Because the disinfectant softens the brush bristles, restore hardness to them by soaking for fifteen minutes in a fifty percent salt and water solution.

EXERCISE REQUIREMENTS

There is a difference between *exercising* your horse and *working* him. Exercise maintains the body's fitness: work develops the talents of the

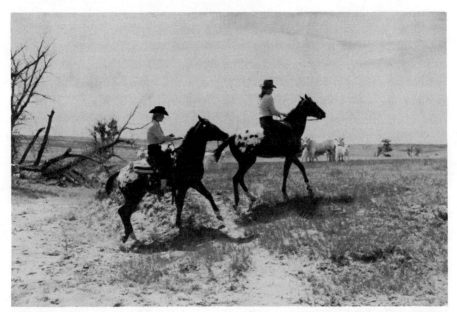

Figure 60. Pleasure riding is as much a part of a horse's education as ring schooling.

horse. Before being put to work, the horse must be fit enough physically and mentally to effortlessly maintain his exercise time without fatigue. Only then can work time be instituted and gradually increased. If pushed into work before he's fit from exercise, or left for days without work and then ridden hard, your horse is very susceptible to injury.

To get an adult riding horse into condition takes about a month and a half—a minimum of thirty minutes daily at the walk and trot to start, with fifteen minutes of cantering added after a few days. This program is based on the horse being ridden six days a week. The ideal amount of exercise per day is forty-five minutes morning and night, regardless of whether the horse is boarded or kept in pasture. After the horse is sufficiently fit, riding time can be increased fifteen minutes per week for work requirements.

At the point of peak conditioning, your horse should be able to be exercised thirty minutes and worked thirty minutes, on the flat at one session without fatigue. Since each horse has it own schooling limitations, depending on use, age, health, and conformation, there are no hard, set rules for time. Your common sense and a knowledge of schooling goals should allow you to set guidelines. The following points may make it easier for you to set these time and task limits.

1. An extended gait over a period of time tires the horse and should only be used for schooling, not as a pleasure gait.

2. The working trot, which is about 9 mph, is easier on the horse than a canter. It should not, however, be used exclusively to cover ground. Alternate it with the walk and canter to avoid tiring the animal.

3. Any new or old maneuvers in schooling will be better accepted if they're practiced for a short time to avoid overstressing the mind and body. New maneuvers should be introduced after firmly established moves are practiced, and terminated on a successful note. Never let the horse feel as though he's failed. End the schooling session with a good feeling of success and the horse will be more likely to work well for you the next day.

4. Strenuous exercise or work, unless the horse is fit, can damage the lungs. At a working trot the horse uses four times as much air as when he's standing, and twelve times more when galloping. The wind must therefore be developed along with the mind and the body.

5. Mental fatigue and boredom set in rapidly when the horse is young, green, or already proficient. Overdoing one gait or maneuver can sour the horse and delay future progress. Vary the schooling routine and supplement it with pasture leisure and trail riding.

6. To avoid upsetting your horse mentally, use long, slow canters to build up wind, rather than short gallop sprints. If excitement or

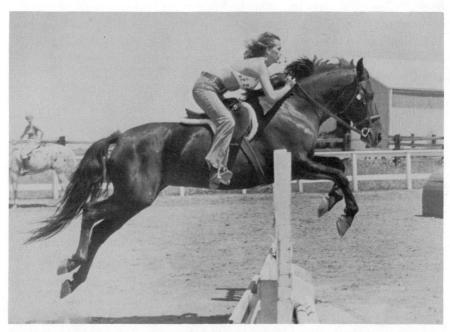

Figure 61. Jumping should be kept to a minimum on schooled horses and those in training. It creates more joint stress than galloping a horse and is a major causative of numerous foot and leg problems.

labored breathing are noted, reduce the pace. Fast trots should also be avoided in excitable horses in favor of long, slow trots.

7. School your horse to use his body. This means work in circles, on poll and jaw flexion, and transitions in gaits and pace. There's less chance of the horse injuring himself if you both know collection and he knows how to use his body.

8. When jumping, don't start until the thirty minutes of exercise time are completed and then, only if the horse is moving without stiffness and with a calm attitude. No horse under three years of age should be jumped consistently over fences or over more than two-and-a-half-foot fences because of the danger of joint damage. When you start over fences—preferably at four years of age—spend a lot of time with ground poles and small fences.

An older or well-schooled jumper will benefit from no more than once or twice a week. During the show season, this work is usually done at the show or once during the week before the show. With an older horse schooling regularly over three-foot fences, limit jumps to twelve to fifteen fences three times per week.

9. Feed according to the amount of work you do and gradually increase feed or supplements as the work increases. Your feeding and nutrition program should be planned with the advice of a professional trainer or your veterinarian to fully meet the horse's needs.

10. The purpose of conditioning a horse is to tone the muscles with slow work and then build wind and fitness with gradual fast work. A conditioning schedule should therefore begin months in advance of the show or hunt season.

Riding Alternatives

When you can't ride your horse, use the alternative of ponying from another horse, longing, swimming, or turning out. Don't run your horse when he's turned out as there is not enough time for a sufficient warmup period and thus, the horse can easily pull or tear a muscle, ligament, or tendon.

Stallion and Mare Exercise

A stallion should be ridden a minimum of thirty minutes a day during the breeding season. The pace should be smooth and relaxed. Daily access to pasture is also necesary for his mental and physical conditioning.

Pregnant mares may be ridden daily, without strenuous exercise, until a few weeks before foaling. This general rule should be checked with your veterinarian due to the possibility of causing the mare to abort if she has difficulty foaling or keeping a foal.

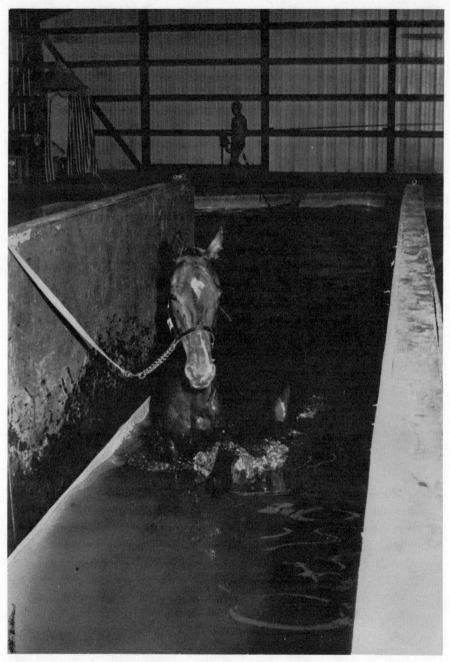

Figure 62. Swimming builds wind and muscles while eliminating the stress on joints that results from working out on hard ground.

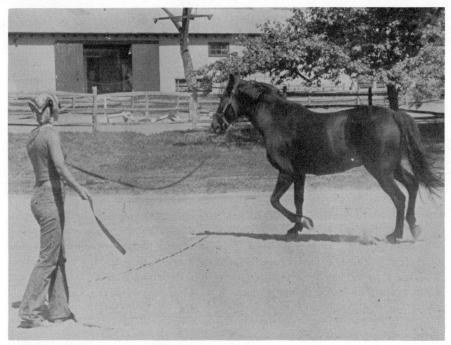

Figure 63. Longeing is an excellent form of exercise when the horse cannot be ridden or is in schooling.

STALL MANAGEMENT

Stalls are necessary evils for horses without pasture access or for those required to be in blemish-free show condition. To make the horse's confinement time more comfortable and less boring, allow him a 12 x 12 box with an outside view, good ventilation, hygienic conditions, and stallmates. Tie stalls are unacceptable for twenty-four hours a day. They allow no freedom for movement, and thereby contribute to foot and leg problems. They're also dangerous should the horse lie down and become cast.

Flooring and Bedding

A stall floor can be concrete, wood, or dirt, with a layer of bedding over it. *Concrete* is not acceptable, since it's too cold during the winter and too hard for the horse's legs. *Wood* is popular when used with shavings and sawdust—moreso than with straw—but absorbs urine and can retain an ammonia smell when nor cleaned daily or treated periodically with lime. Wood also has a tendency to rot and splinter with neglect, age, and pawing. *Dirt* or *clay* is a good floor for use with any type bedding.

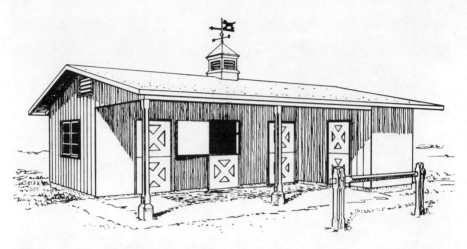

Figures 64 and 65. Blueprint for a functional and easily maintained two- or three-stall barn. The tack room can share space with feed or be eliminated if an extra stall is needed. Be sure to remove the concrete floor from the feed room when converting it into a stall.

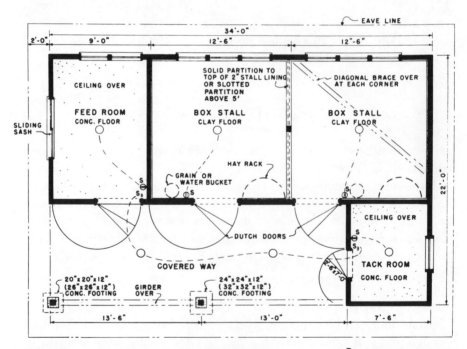

When leveled and spread with lime about six times a year, it will remain relatively maintainance free and hygienic.

Sawdust, as a bedding choice, is absorbent, but may cause respiratory problems, a dirty coat, dry feet, and often, an allergic skin reaction. *Shavings* are slightly less absorbent, but do not ball up in the feet and

94

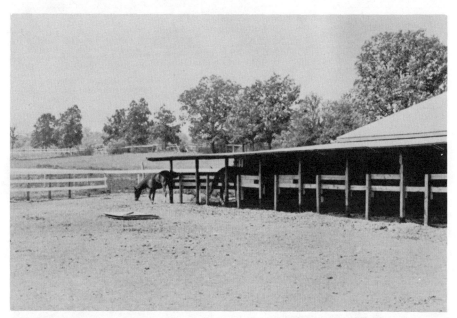

Figure 66. A set-up such as this pasture and stall combination is an economical and healthy way to house a large number of horses.

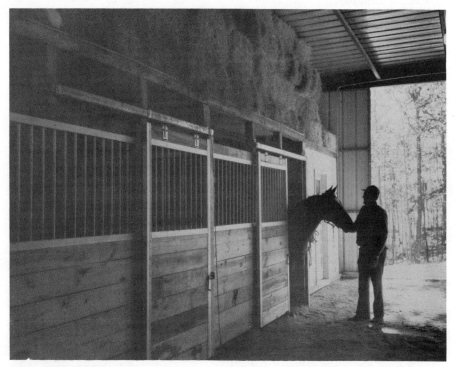

Figure 67. Well-constructed barn with quality sliding doors and hay stored over stalls to save space.

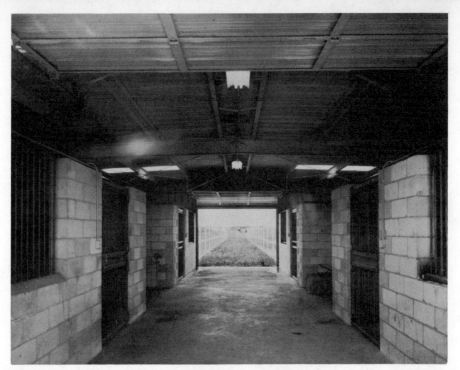

Figure 68. This concrete barn is easy to maintain, virtually fireproof, and cool in the summer.

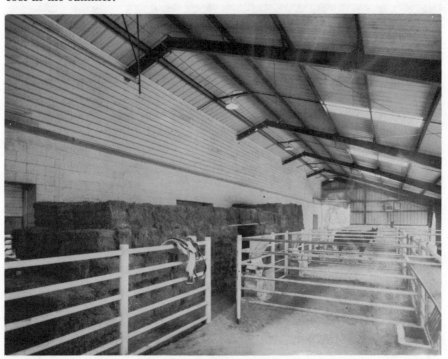

Figure 69. Ideal for hot weather climates, this barn gives horses shelter from rain, but access to fresh air. Use of metal poles instead of boards minimizes maintenance of stalls.

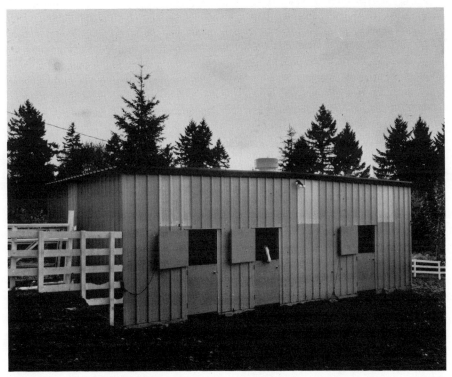

Figure 70. This six-stall barn provides horses with adequate shelter in all temperatures while giving them access to fresh air and pasture.

withdraw as much moisture as sawdust. They also keep the coat cleaner and eliminate many of the breathing problems caused by sawdust. When you buy shavings, get the chips from seasoned wood and check them for unwanted chunks of wood.

Sand is popular in various sections of the country, since it makes a soft bedding. Unfortunately, it holds a lot of moisture and remains wet under the horse. *Straw* makes a clean, soft bed if used in sufficient quantity and kept meticulously picked out. Once the stalks have been broken by the tramping of the horse's feet, they become absorbent and retain both moisture and odor. For best results when using straw, buy it chopped and change it often so the urine drains down through it, rather than being trapped in the broken stalks.

How much bedding to use depends largely on your finances. Ideally, a four-inch depth of shavings or sawdust and two to three bales of straw per week will suffice. When using sand, lay it down at about a three- to four-inch level.

When you clean the stall, pick up the manure first before locating the urine spot. Most horses urinate in the same spot in their stall, so

97

locating it after the first few times will not present a problem. Dig into the wet spot to remove all damp material and repack it with bedding. If mucked out daily, the characteristic ammonia smell of poorly kept stalls will not present a problem.

Disposing of manure depends on where you live. It can be commercially hauled away, dumped away from the stable to decompose, or plowed immediately into a field. If you have a manure pile, keep it away from the water supply and put a foundation of concrete or plastic sheeting under it (Fig. 71).

Tethering and Hobbling

Many owners with a shortage of pasture space stake or tie their animals in the yard or in a grassy area next to the road. This is a dangerous and unwise practice even when safety precautions are taken (Fig. 72).

If you're forced to *tether* your horse, take a chain or nylon rope and cover it with a garden hose to avoid tangling the horse in the line. Be sure the animal is trained to ground tether and won't fight the pull when he feels resistance against his desire to extend grazing limits. Tie away from buildings and farm machinery, and never tie next to the road. Use a heavy nylon halter, not a breakable leather one, and don't tie the rope around the horse's neck.

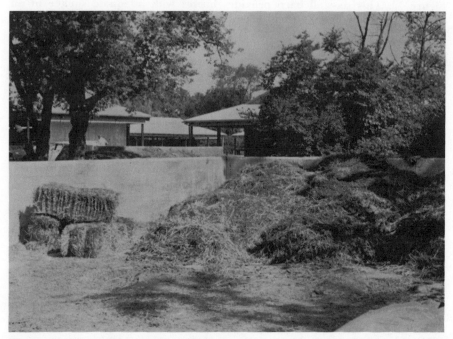

Figure 71. Concrete container for manure is easily maintained and nicer looking than a pile behind a barn.

98

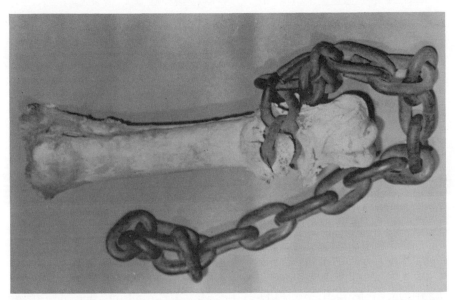

Figure 72. This is a front cannon bone of a horse tethered with a chain that was never removed. As the horse matured from a foal, the chain imbedded itself and the bone grew around it.

When you stake a horse in the yard, sink a heavy-duty twelve-inch tether screw with a large eye ring on it. Use a snap at the end of the tether line to secure it to the screw eye.

Hobbles are for professional use with well-trained horses. Never attempt to use them on your horse unless you have expert guidance. If a horse fights them or panics, he'll usually go down and may cripple himself in the struggle to regain his footing.

Feeding Management

Feeding amounts and types, plus the advisability of vitamin-mineral supplementation present a problem to most nonprofessional horse-owners. The more questions you ask about the subject, the more you'll find that there are a multitude of feeding theories, myths, and dangers involved in the simple process of keeping your horse on a well-balanced and filling diet.

For the horse summered on good pasture, needs are usually met by high-quality grass and water. For winter months, though, and for those periods when the horse is worked, he needs more. To keep him going, you must give concentrates (grains or pellets), hay, and mineralized salt. In addition to these extras, you should also keep in mind that if the feed-stuffs are low in proteins and vitamins and minerals, you must also give a daily nutritive supplement.

Knowing just how much of each to give your horse can determine how well he'll work, breed, and stay healthy. While it's impossible in such a short section of the book to formulate an adequate diet to meet the needs of every age, sex, and work use of horse, there are some guidelines to follow for an average daily ration.

1. Keep in mind that the horse's stomach is small—capable of holding about four gallons—so it's better to feed three to four small feedings rather than one to two large ones.

2. Measure your grain and hay in pounds, rather than giving grain in quarts and hay by flakes. The reason for this is that a quart of oats weighs about one pound, while the same quart can, filled with corn, weighs one and three quarter pounds. A thin flake of hay weighs about two to three pounds, and a thick flake up to five pounds. The average bale of hay weighs forty-five to fifty pounds.

3. The amount of feed given is based on the scientific nutritional scale that a thousand-pound mature horse needs about 8.4 pounds of total digestible nutrients (TDN) per day for maintenance. Unfortunately, concentrates and hay have only a small percentage of TDN per pound, so you have to feed more to get the TDN level up to 8.4. Hays

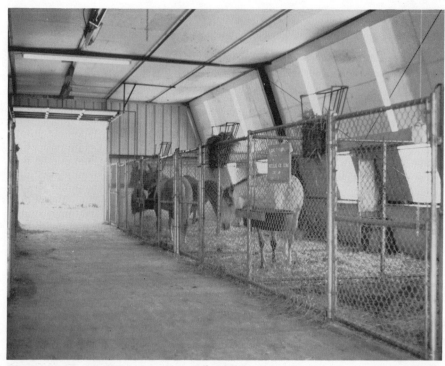

Figure 73. Overhead hay racks and rubber feed tubs meet the demands of convenience, hygiene, and safety within the stall.

average about fifty percent TDN and grains about seventy-five percent TDN.

You, therefore, have to feed about sixteen pounds of hay for maintenance per day (if you feed only hay). If grain is fed with hay, note that since it contains only seventy-five percent TDN, you must give five pounds of grain (yielding four pounds TDN) and nine pounds hay per day (yielding 4.5 pounds TDN) for a light working horse.

4. A boarded horse doing medium work will do well on one pound grain per one hundred pounds body weight and one to one and one quarter pounds hay per one hundred pounds body weight per day.

5. With heavy work, give one and one quarter to one and one half pounds grain and one to one and one quarter pounds hay per hundred pounds body weight per day.

6. Horses in light to heavy work will have more energy and a healthier system if one pound (no more) of protein supplement is given per day with the feed. A protein supplement is a meal of soybean, cottonseed, or linseed. When you start protein supplementation, begin with one quarter pound and work up to one pound in two weeks time.

7. Keep a trace mineralized salt block and clean water available at all times for stall- and pasture-kept horses.

8. A foal can be started on one half pound per hundred pounds body weight of rolled oats at about one month of age. After four to five weeks, increase to one and one half pounds per hundred pounds body weight up to three months of age. By weaning time, consumption should be three to four pounds of concentrate per day.

After weaning, the need for proteins, vitamins, and minerals increases with bone growth. Pasture, plus high-protein concentrate mixtures (about twenty percent protein), is needed. During the winter, give one and one half pounds grain per hundred pounds body weight, and one and one half to two pounds per hundred pound body weight of hay. When hay is high quality, lower the grain poundage and increase the hay.

9. Broodmares should not be allowed to get fat, since it has serious consequences at foaling time due to the large size of the foal and the unfit condition of the mare.

10. Crimping oats increases the nutritive value about five percent. It is also beneficial to feed to horses with poor teeth or to young foals less than 8 months of age. Oats are good for horses in light work, but foals and performance animals need more nutrients than a combination of oats and hay.

11. Corn has less hull than oats, therefore providing less bulk and fiber for digestion. Its high-energy content makes it good for strenuously used horses. Corn is low in protein, and should be fed with a legume hay or protein supplement, particularly when given to broodmares and

growing horses. Molasses can be added to it to reduce dustiness when the corn kernels are rolled and flattened.

12. Molasses is a cheap source of energy. It has a mild laxative effect and should not exceed more than ten to twelve percent of the concentrate ration. When correctly mixed in, you should be able to ball the ration and have it stick together.

13. Commercially prepared rations are available as a complete feed, in hay cube form, or as a combination of roughage and grain in a pellet form. Pellets are easily digestible and contain vitamins and minerals in measured amounts. Many users feel that extra protein supplementation or corn feedings may be necessary for stamina and energy when their horses are strenuously worked.

Nutrients

A *protein* is a complex compound of amino acids needed for body development. The body utilizes it to build and repair tissue and to form bone, blood, skin, hair, and hooves. Especially important to young, growing horses, protein is often given to newborn foals suffering from diarrhea, dehydration, or malnutrition. Protein-rich meals help shed the winter coat and put a bloom on the horse. Take care not to over-proteinize your horse, since proteins can develop body fat.

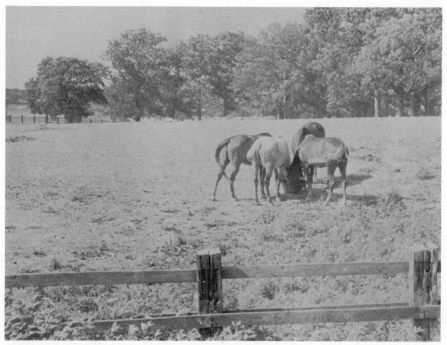

Figure 74. Good pastures, plus additional feed provides a well-balanced diet.

102

Carbohydrates are sugars that constitute the major source of energy. Corn, for example, can contain sixty percent sugar and starch. This is why grains are termed concentrates. If given in excess, fat is deposited on the body.

Vitamins are organic (made from living things) substances used for normal metabolism and growth. When you purchase a commercial preparation for vitamin supplementation, minerals are usually added too. The two elements, however, are different and serve unlike functions in the body. Most vitamins are found in good, green forage, which is why high-quality pasture will supply normal maintenance needs for most horses. For working horses, however, and those still growing or used for breeding, supplementation is a common practice.

Vitamin A requirements can be found in green pasture or early cut alfalfa hay, or good quality mixed hay. Because A is unstable—loses quality—when it is exposed to air and light, it becomes oxidized in five to nine months with normal hay mow storage. If a horse is deficient in vitamin A, the skin, eyes, gut, and respiratory tract are negatively affected. Deficient, pregnant mares abort or bear weak or dead foals. Vitamin A is stored in the liver for three to six months, and if fed at high levels for long periods, can cause vitamin poisoning.

The B-complex vitamins are thiamine (B1), niacin, riboflavin (B2), pyridoxine (B6), pantothenic acid, biotin, choline, folic acid, and B12.

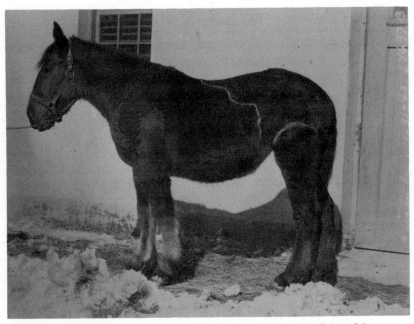

Figure 75. Vitamin A deficiency. Scaly skin outlined in white.

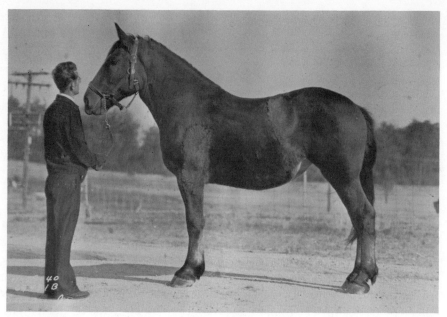

Figure 76. After vitamin A supplementation.

They are obtained from rich pasture, good hay, and brewer's yeast, and are synthesized in the large colon and cecum. These vitamins are necessary for energy and protein metabolism, and a lack may result in loss of appetite, lack of coordination, and anemia.

Vitamin C (ascorbic acid) is assumed by some nutritional studies to be synthesized by the body but not to be required in supplementation. Lack of C has been associated with anemia and poor breeding quality in other studies, however. If the diet you feed is high quality, the horse should not suffer a deficiency.

Vitamin D is synthesized from sun-cured hay and sunshine. During winter months, and where forage is substandard, supplementation is necessary to prevent deficiency. Lack of vitamin D affects skeletal development in young horses and leads to softening of the bones in older ones, particularly when calcium and phosphorus are also deficient. When giving vitamin D supplementation avoid overdoing it, since too much D can lead to deposition of calcium in the tissues and the circulatory system.

Vitamins E and K are both provided by good quality feed and pasture. The daily requirements have not been established, but studies indicate that lack of K has been associated with lack of blood clotting, poor body growth, and loss of function and muscle tone in young and performance horses. Commercial supplementation, under veterinary direction, may prove beneficial in deficiency cases.

Minerals

Minerals are inorganic substances required in small amounts for normal functioning and metabolism. Major minerals found stored in plants and contained in the soil are potassium, chlorine, sodium, calcium, phosphorus, and magnesium. Trace minerals—those found in small quantities—are zinc, manganese, copper, cobalt, iron, and iodine. If your pasture soil is depleted of these, supplementation is necessary for proper body metabolism.

Calcium and phosphorus, along with magnesium, are essential to good bone growth and skeletal maintenance. Forage is high in calcium, and grain high in phosporus. When the body utilizes calcium and phosphorus (Ca:P), it also uses vitamin D to aid absorption and keep the balance between the two minerals. Without this balance, the horse can develop serious skeletal problems. Young horses pushed for growth with a high concentrate ration containing a lot of grain will have enlarged ankles and contracted tendons if not given a calcium supplement or plenty of pasture or hay. Veterinary direction will aid you in keeping an optimal 1:1 balance of Ca:P.

Trace minerals are supplied in most feeds when the soil is good. To ensure against a deficiency, give a trace mineralized salt block or a premix containing these minerals. To avoid toxic oversupplementation, use according to manufacturer's directions.

5

Preventative Medicine and Management

The area of preventative medicine and management deals with the regular care you give to safeguard your horse's health. It includes a periodic and regular worming, shoeing, dental, and immunization program, plus attention to external parasites on the horse and in the stable. Without an effectively planned and executed program of health protection, your horse is very vulnerable to disease, injury, and below-par performance.

Immunization and Tests

1. Encephalomyelitis (Eastern, Western, and Venezuelan strains):
   One or two injections annually depending on vaccine used.

2. Equine Influenza:
   Two injections the first year, four to six weeks apart.
   Yearly booster thereafter for all ages.

3. Tetanus (lockjaw):
   Two injections of tetanus toxoid the first year, four to six weeks apart.
   Yearly booster thereafter for all ages.

4. Strangles:

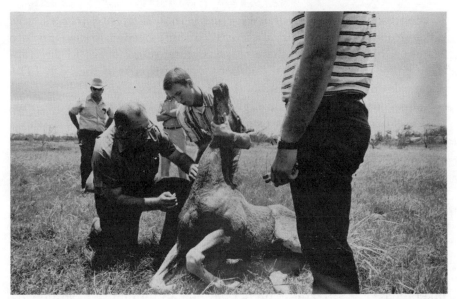

Figure 77. Blood sample being taken from a Texas colt suspected of having VEE.

Immunization is available at the discretion of your veterinarian.

5. A.G.I.D. (Coggins) Test:
   This test is for equine infection anemia (swamp fever). If your horse has a negative test and is in a closed herd, you need not repeat it annually. Most states require a negative test within six months prior to interstate shipment. Racing associations, show committees, and breeding establishments should be contacted for their test requirements.

6. Rhinopneumonitis:
   Two injections the first year, four to eight weeks apart.
   Yearly booster thereafter.

Internal Parasite Management

In past years, worming took place twice a year: spring and after the first frost in the fall to control *bots, ascarids, strongyles, pinworms,* and *stomach worms.* When *tapeworms* were found present, additional treatment for these parasites was given. Today, the practice to effectively control internal parasites is with a regular, consistent program of tube worming— spring and fall—supplemented by a broad-spectrum wormer (called an anthelminthic) in the feed every other month.

107

The reason for more regular worming is that different parasites have different life cycles and varying lengths of time needed to develop into mature adults. The horse, therefore, has many stages of worm development going on at one time throughout different parts of the body. The chemicals in the anthelminthic that kill adults in the intestine will not affect larvae migrating through other parts of the body. So administration of periodic doses of a wormer are needed to kill the newly matured adults and gradually reduce the number of parasites.

Once parasitic infestation is under control, you don't stop worming. Horses are constantly reinfested by ingesting eggs and infective larvae in bedding, grass, and manure. Thus, you must continue worming to prevent a buildup of parasites (Fig. 78).

Strongyles

Strongyles (bloodworms) are the most serious internal parasites and can cause severe internal injury, and sometimes death due to heavy infestations (Fig. 79). Horses do not develop an immunity to strongyles, which can be classified into strongyles (three species) and small strongyles (about forty species).

Within the *large strongyles* group are *S. vulgaris, S. equinus,* and *S. edentatus.* The former is more common to most states.

The life cycle of *S. vulgaris* begins when the horse swallows the larvae

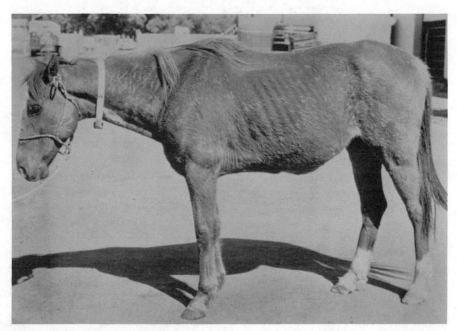

Figure 78. Unthrifty appearance due to parasitic infestation.

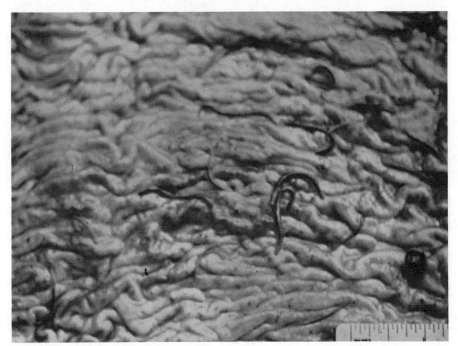

Figure 79. Large strongyles.

clinging to pasture grass or bedding. There then follows a long migration of the larval developmental stages through the horse's internal organs, especially within the walls of mesenteric arteries. This larval migration causes subsequent severe tissue damage and bleeding. While the larvae migrate, they feed on tissue, so blood clots form around the injured area. These frequently break off and plug arteries. The results of heavy migration are colic, lameness, and digestive problems.

When the larvae finish their migration through arteries and tissues, they return to the cecum and colon of the large intestine to mature and lay eggs. During the adult stage they attach to the intestine lining and suck blood. The eggs pass from the body in the horse's feces and hatch outside the horse, where infestation again takes place when the horse eats infected grass or bedding.

Strongyle control is difficult, because the larvae can't be affected by chemicals during their migratory stages. Larval development takes about six months, so a good worming program is important to control strongyle buildup.

The migratory phase of small strongyles (Fig. 80) is much simpler, since their activity is usually limited to the gut wall. Some small strongyles *encyst* (form nodules) in the mucous membrane lining of the cecum, while others remain unattached in the large intestine. While

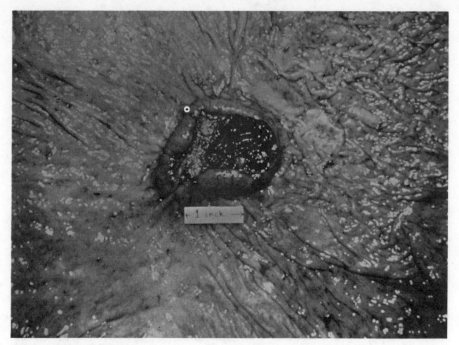

Figure 80. Small strongyles.

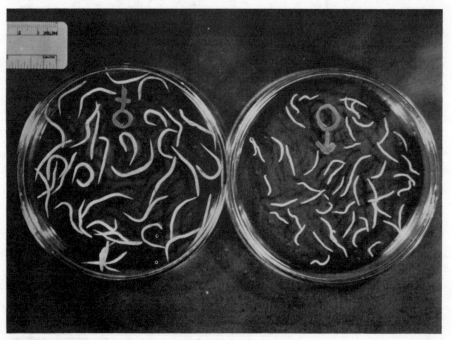

Figure 81. Pinworms.

encysted, chemical treatment is ineffective. Unlike the lengthy development period of large strongyles, the small worms take approximately six to twelve weeks to develop from larvae to adults.

Depending on the number of larvae present in the cecum, ruptures of the nodules create sores and ulcerations that can lead to hemorrhage and impairment of the organ's function. The digestive ability of the large intestine, if there's heavy parasitic infestation, is also impaired and diarrhea or constipation can develop.

The reproductive capacity of small strongyles can be up to twenty-five million eggs per day. Even with good management procedures such as pasture rotation and proper manure disposal, strongyle control relies mainly on the use of anthelminthics. These drugs kill the adults in the intestine, thus breaking up the reproductive cycle.

Pinworms

There are two species of pinworms (Fig. 81) found in the horse's large intestine, the *common pinworm* and the *minute pinworm*. The adult female common pinworm lives in the colon of the gastrointestinal tract and deposits eggs around the anus. The intense irritation caused by this procedure causes the horse to rub its hindquarters, thereby giving the tail a ratty appearance.

Once the eggs leave the body, they can survive for long periods of time in water, or adhere to fences, grass, bedding, and walls. Infestation begins when the eggs are ingested and the larvae develop into adults—a time period of about five months.

The life cycle of the minute pinworm is carried out entirely in the horse's large intestine. There is no five month wait to become sexually mature, because the adult females produce offspring that are sexually mature when they hatch. Contamination from one horse to another occurs when fresh feces are eaten. To break the transmission chain, a regular worming program is necessary.

Ascarids

Ascarid (roundworm) infection is more common to horses under a year of age, as acquired resistance to infection seems to develop as the animal matures. Adult ascarids (Fig. 82) live in the small intestine and produce about two hundred thousand eggs per female per day. The eggs pass in the feces and develop into larvae in about two weeks. Unlike the strongyles, which hatch outside the body, ascarids remain in a shell for years until they're ingested.

They hatch in the intestine and migrate through the wall and on to the liver and lungs. In the lungs, they break through the capillaries and go into the respiratory passages where they're coughed up and swallowed a

111

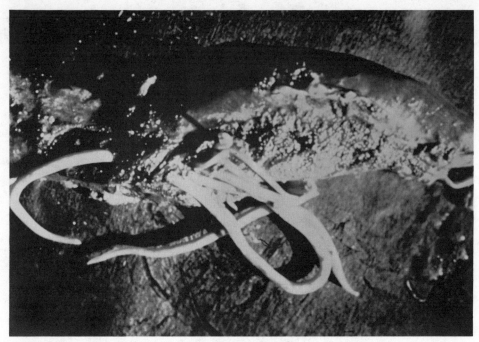

Figure 82. Ascarids.

second time. Then they pass into the small intestine where ten weeks are spent reaching the adult stage. The entire process from ingestion to adult takes about three months to complete.

Roundworm migration damages the liver and lungs and causes rupture of the intestine in some horses, particularly weanlings in the fall of the year. In addition to this damage, ascarid infestation causes a potbelly look, rough coat, impaired growth, colic, and diarrhea.

Botfly

Bots are present in almost every age horse kept on full or part-time pasture. The two most prevalent of three botfly species are *Gastrophilus intestinalis* and *G. nasalis*. Both produce one generation per year and lay the eggs on the horse's leg hairs. When the horse itches or rubs its legs with its mouth, the warmth and rubbing action causes the eggs to hatch on the lips.

After hatching, the larvae enter the mouth and burrow into the tongue and oral tissues. After about three weeks, they pass to the stomach (Fig. 83) and remain for up to ten months before detaching and passing out in the feces.

Damage is most severe in the stomach, since deep pits (Fig. 84) develop at points of larval attachment. Problems such as colic and digestive disorders and obstructions occur with heavy infestations. In many cases of

112

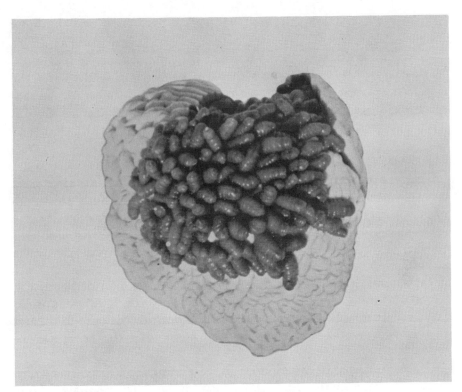

Figure 83. Heavy infestation of stomach bots.

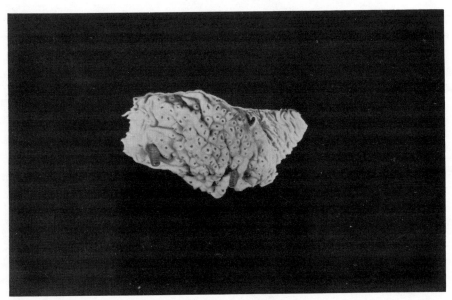

Figure 84. Bots attached to stomach lining. Note holes in lining where bots have eaten into stomach.

heavy larval infestation, the stomach wall is perforated and the horse dies.

To control bots, begin in the summer with removal of the nits (eggs) by shaving the legs or sponging with warm water to artificially hatch the eggs. While these measures minimize chances of infection, broad-spectrum drugs for bots should be administered at the same time as anthelminthics for strongyle control.

Tapeworms

The *tapeworm* specie that is found most frequently in the intestinal tract is *Anoplocephala perfoliata*. About one to two inches in length, this tape-worm clusters in the cecum and produces severe ulcerations of the membrane. If there's a heavy buildup, the horse has digestive problems and lack of vitality. A second specie, infrequently found, measures twelve inches and develops in the rear half of the intestine.

Tapeworms spend part of their life cycle in an intermediate host, the orbatid mite, which lives in woods and pastures. It takes approximately three months for the encysted tapeworm to leave the mite, and another two months to develop into an adult after the horse has ingested it.

Unless you or your veterinarian have reason to suspect tapeworm infection, it's not routine to check for them. If, however, you have a large mite population in your geographical area, one or two yearly fecal checks will ascertain the presence of tapeworms.

Stomach Worms

Stomach worms are carried to the horse by an intermediate host, the fly. If the worms gain access to the horse's stomach, the larvae develop into adults, which colonize and produce stomach abscesses. Often, though, the larvae are deposited in wounds where they cause summer sores. When deposited in the eye, they'll cause conjunctivitis. The three species of stomach worms found in horses respond to some drugs used for strongyle control, but those deposited in other external areas need veterinary treatment and external care.

EXTERNAL PARASITES

Mites

Mites are small, almost invisible parasites (Fig. 85) that cause an itchy, contagious disease known by several names—mange, scabies, scab, or itch. Several types of mange occur in horses, but the ones produced

114

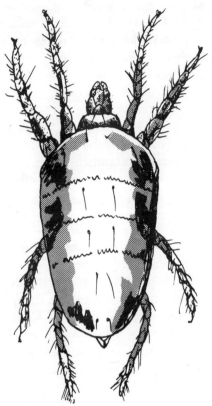

Figure 85. Mite.

by the *sarcoptic mite* and the *psoroptic mange mite* are the most troublesome and contagious.

The sarcoptic mange mite burrows through the skin and secretes an irritating substance that causes hairless lesions in irregular patches. The scabs that develop at the center of each small patch are caused by a discharge that forms over the burrowing mite. As the mites burrow, eggs are laid under the skin and hatch into larval mites that mature in two weeks or so.

When the irritation from borrowing and secreting the toxic substance becomes intense, the horse rubs the infected areas. The skin becomes abraded and large scabs are formed. Eventually the skin dries and takes on a thickened, wrinkled appearance. When this happens, secondary bacterial infections usually occur.

Psoroptic mange is caused by mites that bite the skin and suck blood, but do not burrow. This type of mange is more contagious than sarcoptic mange, since the mite live on the skin and feed on the horse's serum and lymph.

The appearance of psoroptic lesions is usually under the mane and forelock, and around the tail. Unlike the dry scabs of sarcoptic mange, the lesions remain moist and enlarge as the mites increase their periphery of biting and sucking activity. Hair loss follows and like the other mange form, the skin wrinkles, itching is intense, and scabs cover the infected area.

Treatment for mange is a combination of quarantine and spraying with a chemical mite solution. In some areas, horses are dipped to control mites. In herds where only a few animals are infected, the entire herd should be sprayed. Veterinary recommendation for treatment is usually two applications at a two-week interval.

Ticks

Throughout the United States are many species of ticks that reduce the horse's vitality because they cause blood loss and skin irritation. Death is not uncommon in cases of heavy, uncontrolled infestation.

Some of the better known ticks are the Rocky Mountain spotted fever tick (a possible carrier of Western equine encephalitis); the tropical horse tick; the spinose ear tick; and the Gulf Coast tick.

There are many more species of biting and sucking ticks indigenous to specific parts of the country, and they all have the same thing in common. They're hard to eradicate from an area and they do considerable damage to the horse if not treated promptly.

Ticks begin their life cycle as eggs and larvae on the ground. Once the ticks reach the larval stage, they crawl onto vegetation and await a host. It takes about a week or more for the larvae to metamorphose into an eight-legged nymph that sucks blood for some six months. Then the nymph drops to the ground where it matures into an adult. Eggs are

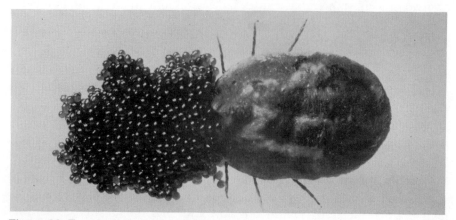

Figure 86. Female tick laying eggs.

116

laid (Fig. 86), and the cycle repeats itself. The female tick dies after the eggs are laid.

Ticks are capable of living many months before finding a host. This is why you can have a tick-free herd infected quickly when you move the horses into a vacant pasture in tick country. Some foresight as to pasture, stall, and shelter spraying will greatly reduce the number of ticks.

For animals already infected, dipping is effective for large numbers of horses. Individual animals can be dusted or sprayed to guard against infestation. To remove ticks, light a match, blow it out, and touch the hot end to the bottom of the tick or just behind its embedded head. Avoid pulling the body away with tweezers, since the mouthpiece will remain in the skin and cause irritation.

Lice

The biting and sucking species of lice (Fig. 87) produce severe itching and subsequent biting and rubbing of the affected areas by the horse. Without prompt treatment, these spots become raw, hairless, and susceptible to secondary bacterial infection. Weight loss is noticeable, particularly in the young and aged horse. An unthrifty appearance is also common.

The *sucking louse* spends its entire life cycle on the horse. Eggs are laid in the hair and develop in two weeks. The young then commence to feed on the horse's blood. During their rapid growth period, anemia can develop. The *biting louse* does not pierce the skin, but instead, feeds on hair and skin flakes. The life cycle from egg to louse is essentially the same.

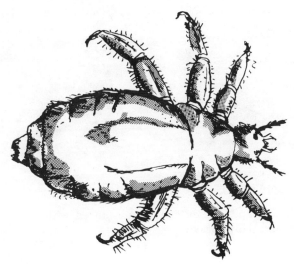

Figure 87. Louse.

117

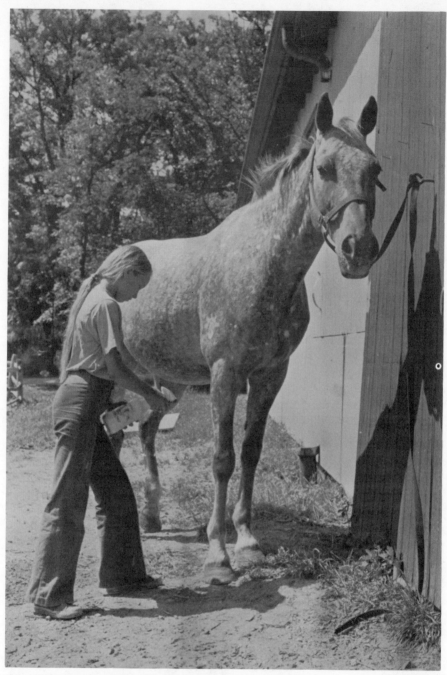

Figure 88. Irritation and disease can be minimized with a good fly irradication program and daily spraying.

To control lice, ask your veterinarian for a powder spray without an oil base (it burns the coat) and spray both the animal and its living quarters. If you clip the coat before spraying, burn the hair and disinfect all utensils with the spray. Extreme sanitary measures should be taken with all tack and grooming equipment, since biting lice can survive without a host for about ten to thirty days if they're attached to hair in blankets or combs.

Mosquitoes

Mosquitoes can be a major cause of death and injury to horses, not only because of the irritation they cause, but because at least eight species are capable of transmitting equine encephalomyelitis. These insects can't be eliminated entirely, but there are many management techniques available to reduce their numbers.

Keep your horse immunized annually for all encephalomyelitis strains. Next, keep your stable animals lightly blanketed in the summer, and screen all doors and windows. Pasture-kept horses should be sprayed or wiped regularly with a commercial antimosquito solution (Fig.88).

The most effective management technique is to contact your local mosquito abatement and control agency for assistance and advice peculiar to your water and land. Effective control hinges on understanding the life cycle and breaking it.

Basically it takes four stages to complete the cycle: eggs, larva, pupa, and adult. The eggs are laid on water in masses of one hundred to four hundred and hatch in a day or two into wiggling larvae. The larvae molt into a pupa, and the pupa develops into a mosquito in a few days. The male mosquito is harmless and prefers the juices of vegetation, unlike the female's preference for nourishment.

Since it takes only a week to complete the egg to adult cycle, the chain can be broken by emptying all water containers or floating a light film of oil on the water's surface. The oil seals off the breathing tubes of the larvae and pupae. Some states permit the use of mosquito fish, *Gambusia affins*, to eat the larvae as they hatch. These fish are extremely effective in controlling mosquito production in ponds and lakes. While there are many chemicals available that are fast acting, check the brand with the abatement agency to see that it is not a hazard for fish or wildlife.

Flies

Houseflies, stable flies, blackflies, horseflies, sand flies, blowflies, and gnats all make horses and owners miserable. They lower vitality through constant biting, cause weight loss, affect performance, and may stunt growth in young horses.

To reduce the fly population, keep up a regular chemical spraying

119

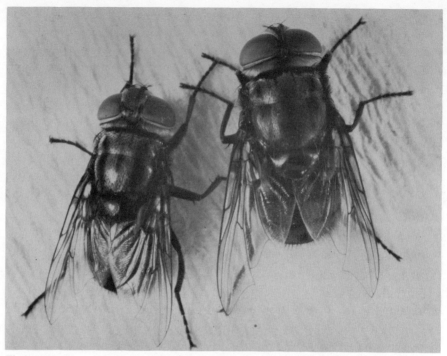

Figure 89. Screwworm flies lay eggs around open wounds. The larvae burrow into the wounds to feed on living flesh. Left untreated, death can result.

schedule for the barn, in addition to removal or proper disposal of manure. Screen all entrances to the stable, and blanket your horse with a fly sheet.

CARE AND DISEASES OF THE MOUTH

A yearly veterinary examination of the teeth and mouth is important to your horse's health and comfort while being worked and for proper mastication of food.

The Teeth

There are four types of teeth in the horse's mouth, depending on his age and sex. In the adult male and female are twelve *incisors*, top and bottom, which form the central, middle, and laterals. At the back of the mouth are twenty-four grinding *cheek teeth*, top and bottom.

The adult also has up to two *wolf teeth*, which are vestiges of prehistoric premolars. These small teeth are located in front of the upper cheek teeth and are usually removed because they can interfere with the bit and cause pain. In the adult male (seldom in the female) are four additional small teeth called *canines* or *tusks*. They're located in the middle of the bars, on the top and bottom. These are not usually removed, since they seldom interfere with the bit's action.

Horses need to have their cheek teeth *floated* or filed down once a year. This is because the grinding action of the teeth causes the inside edges of the lower cheek teeth and the outside edges of the upper ones to become sharp and irritating to the tongue and cheek. Once these are scratched or cut, the horse cannot chew properly and will drop food in partially ground clumps.

There are several congenital conditions of the mouth that cannot be corrected by dental work, but should be watched due to possible mouth damage and eating interference.

The first of these is *parrot mouth* (Fig. 90), in which the upper incisors jut out and overlap the lower incisors. Because the upper teeth are not ground down with normal use, they grow longer and can prevent the horse from grasping food. Dental rasping of the lower and upper incisors

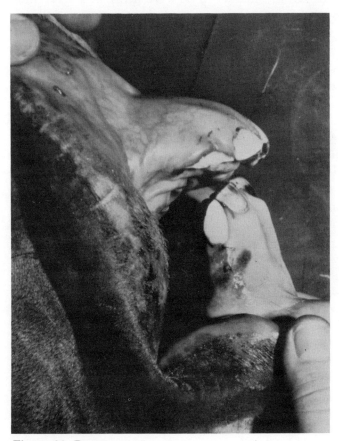

Figure 90. Parrot mouth.

and cheek teeth is recommended to keep the horse from losing weight.

Another congenital deformity is the *undershot jaw*. Here the lower incisors are longer and overlap the upper ones. Treatment consists of shortening the incisors and keeping the cheek teeth level.

Irregularities in the wearing surface of the teeth are termed a *wave-formed mouth*. When there's irregularity in height, the term *step-formed mouth* is used. Both are kept in check by rasping down sharp edges and giving a suitable diet for each condition. When a horse has no irregularities, the condition is called a *smooth mouth*. It results from an equal wearing of the enamel and dentine of each tooth and may occur in youngsters as a dental structure defect. In older animals it develops when the tooth crown becomes worn to the root. There is no dental treatment for a smooth mouth, only a diet that is easily chewed.

Another condition that cannot be satisfactorily treated is *shear mouth* (Fig. 91). The upper cheek teeth grow outside of the lower ones and overlap like scissor blades. The constant wearing action of one set against the other causes the enamel to be worn away and leaves the teeth very sharp. Periodic rasping and a soft diet are recommended.

The Mouth

Excessive salivation or *slobbering* may stem from inflammation of the mouth, abnormal teeth conditions, or the presence of a foreign object in the mouth. It is also known to occur following the administration of certain drugs. Slobbering, in some horses, is caused by an obstruction or paralysis of the pharynx or esophagus, thereby inhibiting the natural swallowing reflex. Salivation noted during riding or driving highly collected horses is the result of keeping the neck in such a position that saliva can't be swallowed.

Treatment consists of finding and removing the cause. If the slobbering is medically correctible, the condition will disappear in time. If, however,

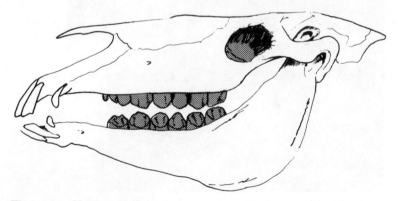

Figure 91. Shear mouth.

122

it's produced by improper bitting or handling, the horse may discontinue salivating only with proper schooling.

Tongue inflammation, or *glossitis*, is a common occurrence in the horse and one of the easiest to overlook when feeding and bitting problems occur. The tongue can be injured by a severe bit, splinters, irritating substances such as an antichew wood solution, sharp teeth, and careless handling of the tongue during an examination. If the swelling is severe, the horse carries the tongue between its front teeth and may accidentally bite it while eating.

Treatment consists of finding the cause and giving an antiseptic mouthwash for wounds. A soft diet while the tongue is healing is recommended.

CARE OF THE FEET

The hoof wall, like your fingernail, is composed of dead skin cells that are pushed down from a bed of living cells. In the horse, this bed is the coronary band. As explained in the first chapter, the hoof wall grows at about three eighths of an inch per month and must be kept trimmed periodically.

Some horses ridden on sandy or hard ground will keep their feet worn

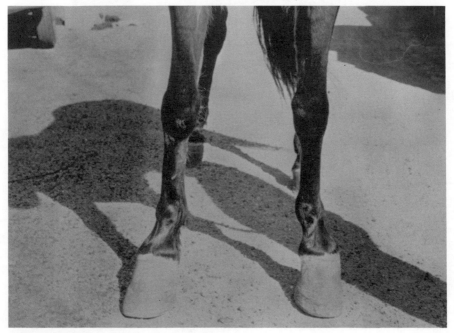

Figure 92. Long overdue for shoeing.

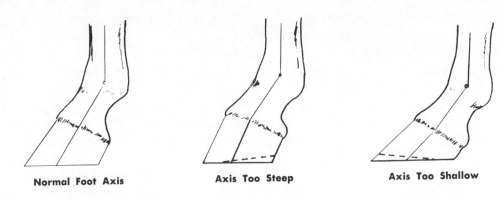

Normal Foot Axis   **Axis Too Steep**   **Axis Too Shallow**

Figure 93. Angles of the foot.

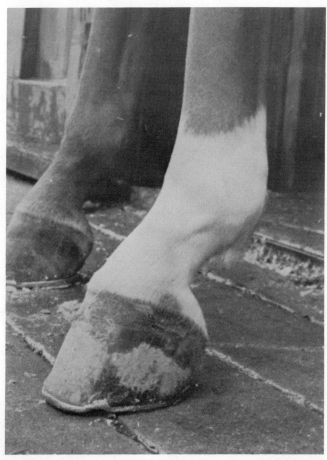

Figure 94. A poor shoeing job. The foot angle is broken and places stress on the pastern area.

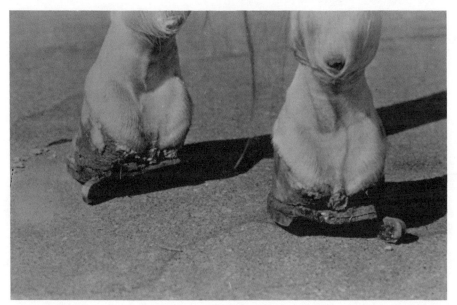

Figure 95. Corrective shoeing can aid interference and striding problems. These are rear shoes with pads and outside trailer calks.

to a length that requires only occasional trimming and rasping. For most others, though, the foot needs the attention of a farrier every six to eight weeks (Fig 92). From age one month, a horse needs competent work on his feet to give them a correct angle and length, and to correct or alter problems. With early care, significant conformation alterations can be performed and future foot problems nipped in the bud.

Foot Angle

The angle of the foot—about fifty degrees in the front and five degrees higher in the rear—determines the *path of flight* (Fig. 93). This is the arch of the foot during a stride. With a normal angle, the foot makes a semicircular arc. When a horse is conformed with a short, upright foot, he breaks over quicker and is at his highest point in the stride during the last half of the stride. When the hooves are long and sloping and there is less of an angle, the highest stride point occurs right after the foot leaves the ground. Since it takes longer for the foot to break over here, the stride is longer and the contact with the ground more gentle and less traumatic than with an upright angle.

The farrier can lengthen the short arc a bit more and shorten the lengthy one simply by lowering or raising the heel height. To do this during one shoeing, or to too great an extreme, will produce severe stress on the legs. It's therefore important for you to know your farrier's reputation in corrective shoeing before you ask him to change your horse.

125

6

Diseases of the Head and Body

If you have an elementary, conversant knowledge of the more common diseases your horse may develop, you'll be better equipped to spot and handle problems before they become serious. A good foundation in equine diseases also makes understanding your veterinarian's explanation of a problem easier—for both of you.

Colic

The word *colic* refers to mild to severe abdominal pain that can occur once, or become recurrent (chronic). It's one of the major causes of death and should be considered a situation needing immediate veterinary attention.

Symptoms of colic can vary with the severity of the pain, or the cause of the intestinal problem. The horse usually is found circling the stall, pawing at the ground, looking at or biting his flanks, sweating, rolling, or having an elevated heart rate of eighty to one hundred beats per minute or higher. When you see any of these signs, call your veterinarian. If the animal is *resting* quietly, stay with him and keep him warm: don't walk him for hours. Walk the horse that is down and thrashing or on his feet and violently distressed. Then stop and rest if he's quiet.

With *spasmodic colic*, you can hear loud intestinal rumbling. With *flatulent colic*, rumblings are slight, but the stomach is distended with

126

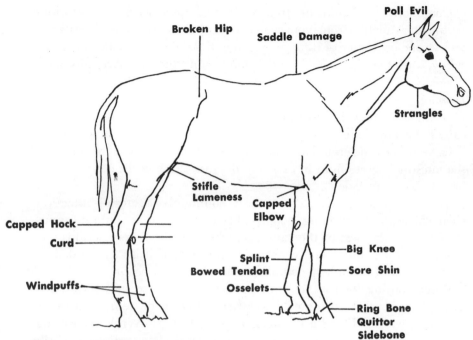

Figure 96. Disease and injury sites.

gas, and high pitched gassy "pings" are heard. A third type, called *impaction*, offers little or no sound because neither food nor gas is being pushed through the intestines.

Colic can be caused by parasitic infestation, due to migration damage from the strongyle larvae, moldy or spoiled feeds, and inconsistent or incorrect feeding programs. It's also triggered by overfeeding, feeding while hot or tried, overwatering while hot, too much spring grass, ingestion of sand, indigestible hay, or by diseases such as enteritis and purpura hemorrhagica. Impactions can be caused by lack of sufficient water, especially during the winter.

Conjunctivitis

Conjuctivitis is an inflammation of the mucous membranes that line the inner surface of the eyelids (the conjuctiva). It occurs most frequently in the warm months to pastured as well as boarded horses. When dust, pollen, or other irritants get in the eyes, the horse rubs them and irritates the delicate tissues. Then flies congregate around the irritated, weeping eye and introduce bacterial infection into the already inflamed tissues.

When this happens, the eyes tear, the lids swell, and eventually a pus discharge appears. Flies continue to irritate the eye and perpetuate rubbing by the horse.

127

Conjunctivitis should be treated immediately with an antibiotic ointment available from your veterinarian, since continued irritation and secondary injury of the eye is common. While the irritation is subsiding, wash the discharge from the skin around the eye on a daily basis.

Diarrhea

Diarrhea, or enteritis, results from an inflammation of the intestines. It causes the bowel's contents to be forced through faster than normal. Because of the accelerated action of intestinal contractions, the glands of the intestine secrete fluid in excess and cause the bowel's content to be heavily moisture laden.

The precipitating causes are most commonly bacterial infection, chemical or plant poisoning, poor quality feedstuffs that contain fungus, or nerves. Regardless of the cause, diarrhea can be a very serious condition requiring immediate veterinary attention. If it isn't attended to, dehyration and secondary complications are apt to occur.

While waiting for the veterinarian, keep the horse indoors or in a shelter and blanket during cold weather. Offer clean, temperate water and don't withhold food if the horse appears hungry. While recovering, your veterinarian will probably advise several days ration of easily digested food and light work, if any.

Encephalitis

Encephalitis, or sleeping sickness, is an acute viral infection of the brain and spinal cord. Three different strains of virus can cause the disease: Eastern, Western, and Venezuelan (VEE) equine encephalomyelitis viruses. Most horses are afflicted by only one strain, but those animals transported interstate may contract and spread all three strains.

Encephalitis is characterized by depression and fever, in the beginning stage, along with a possible reluctance to move (Fig. 97) and drooping lower lip. Poor coordination and staggering are common in the more advanced stages of the disease.

This disease can be transmitted to humans, but not directly from horses. The chain begins with infected birds that are bitten by mosquitoes, and then to man and horse. The viruses cause inflammation of the brain and spinal cord. Death occurs in about fifty percent of all infected equine cases with some of those that recover being permanently afflicted due to nerve damage.

There is no specific treatment for the disease, therefore bi-annual vaccination is important to prevent sleeping sickness.

Equine Infectious Anemia

Equine infectious anemia (EIA), also called swamp fever, is caused by a

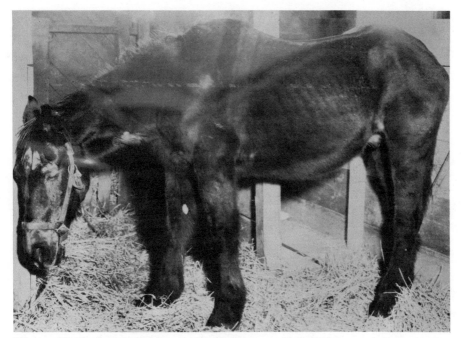

Figure 97. Typical attitude of a horse with encephalitis.

virus found in the blood and tissues of infected animals—and remains there even after recovery. Horses that carry the virus can infect other animals, principally by blood transmission, and less often by discharge from their eyes and nose, stallion's semen and mare's milk, urine and manure. An EIA-AGID (Coggins) diagnostic test is available to detect swamp fever, and is required by most states before the horse can be moved into the state.

EIA appears in an acute form, chronic form, and a carrier stage with no symptoms. In the *acute stage* there is a rise in temperature to 150° or higher with the fever remaining steady or intermittent. The breathing is rapid, depression acute, and the animal generally loses weight (Fig. 98) even though eating continues. Urination is frequent, diarrhea develops with advancement of the disease, and swelling develops on the body and legs. Many horses stagger from weakness or develop hindleg paralysis.

As the disease nears its end, anemia develops and the mucous membranes of the mouth, eyes, and anus pale. The horse's pulse will be noticeably weak and may be accompanied by irregular heart action. In most cases, the symptoms last three to five days in the acute form and may occur several times before the animal dies.

In the *chronic form* of the disease, afflicted horses appear to recover and may live in an emaciated, weakened condition for several years or more. EIA often recurs many times and lasts longer each time until

129

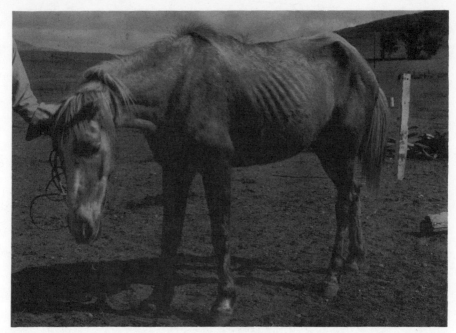

Figure 98. An advanced case of equine infectious anemia that ended with the death of the horse.

death ends it. For the duration of their life, chronically diseased horses are carriers with the potential of infecting healthy horses.

The *carrier form* of infectious anemia is the most dangerous because it has no symptoms. Infected horses carry the virus for their life time and are infectious, even though they've never had an apparent attack of EIA. Some carriers may develop an acute or chronic form after stressful work or transportation, or sickness.

Equine Influenza

Equine influenza is a highly contagious viral disease that produces a cough, high temperature, nasal discharge, weakness, loss of appetite, and general depression. The disease is caused by two viruses that produce identical symptoms, and thus, a horse can contract influenza twice. The viruses are transmitted primarily in sneeze and cough droplets, and indirectly in water, feed, and bedding. Transmission is greatest where large groups of horses are stabled or when horses are worked hard or kept in a poorly managed condition.

Death seldom occurs when a horse is given complete rest, following contraction of influenza, and when secondary bacterial complications do not set in. If the horse is prematurely returned to work, prolongation of symptoms is noticeable.

The best prevention for equine influenza is by regular immunization with a killed vaccine. If a horse in a herd or barn contracts influenza, quarantine the animal immediately until all symptoms disappear. Antibiotic treatment is indicated for fevers over 102°. Antibiotics do not control the effect of the virus on the horse's system—just the secondary bacterial complications.

Equine Viral Rhinopneumonitis

Equine viral rhinopneumonitis is a contagious viral infection that can cause abortion in pregnant mares and upper respiratory infection in younger horses. In some cases, the virus invades the spinal cord and causes incoordination.

Symptoms of this viral disease occur two to ten days after exposure and are characterized by a 102–107° fever that persists up to a week, with a watery nasal discharge. In more severe cases with secondary bacterial infection, the discharge is thick and accompanied by a deep cough and loss of appetite.

To prevent the spread of rhinopneumonitis and its subsequent complications, call your veterinarian when symptoms first appear. Rest, a gradual return to work, and good nursing care are important to recovery. Rhinopneumonitis vaccine is available from your veterinarian.

Facial Paralysis

Facial paralysis is caused by damage to one or, rarely, both of the seventh cranial nerves that run down from the brain, emerge at each ear base, and branch out on the side of the face. These nerves control the movement of the muscles of the ears, eyelids, cheeks, lips, and nostrils. The most frequent cause of damage is an injury, but occasionally the nerve is affected by an abscess following an attack of strangles.

The symptoms of facial paralysis may include a drooping eyelid or lip (Fig. 99), and an inability to lift the ear to an upright position on the affected side. Because of the nerve damage, the horse loses his ability to drink correctly, since his sucking power is limited.

Facial paralysis does not affect the horse's serviceability, but does inhibit certain types of showing. In many cases, time causes the condition to disappear. While there is no effective treatment for this disease, the horse may be made more comfortable by seeing that the halter and bridle fit well, that all food and water are plentiful, and that he is given enough time to consume what he wants.

Heaves

Heaves, or broken wind, is emphysema. Within the lungs are air sacs (alveoli) that become torn and decrease the amount of oxygen capable of

131

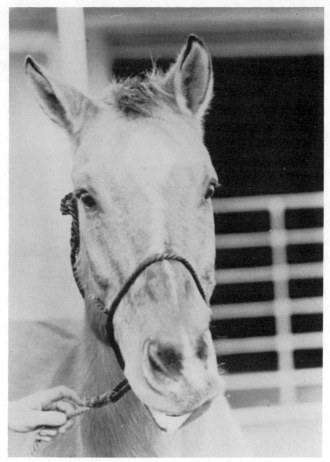

Figure 99. Facial paralysis.

being taken into the lungs. At this point, the horse gasps to fill the lungs and eventually develops a chronic cough characteristic of a heavey horse. The abdominal muscles of the horse contract on each expiration, and a furrow, or heave line, develops in the flanks.

Treatment will not always provide a cure, just relief. If the hay is dampened, coughing may be reduced as dustiness is reduced. Bedding should be changed from dusty shavings to straw, large shavings, or sand—anything that's not dusty. If possible, keep a heavey horse on year-round pasture.

Heaves can possibly be prevented if moldy hay is never fed, bedding watched, and all respiratory problems attended to immediately. Heaves is often attributed to an allergic reaction, a sequel to bronchitis or pneumonia, or chronic coughing due to moldy food or too bulky, dusty food.

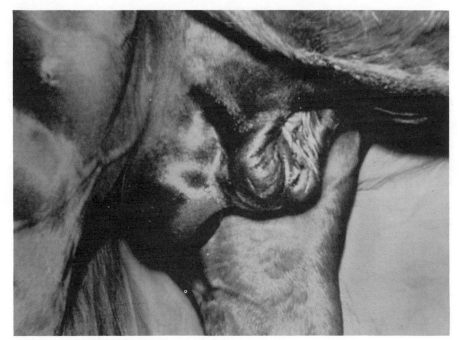

Figure 100. Scrotal hernia in a stallion.

Hernia

A *hernia* is a noticeable swelling occurring at the navel, scrotum (Fig. 100), or flank area. It's caused when the walls containing the internal organs are ruptured and the contents protrude to lie under the skin as a swelling. The cause may be hereditary, congenital, or due to strain or injury.

It is important to have a hernia examined, since a portion of the protruding intestine may become strangulated and cause death. The symptoms of a strangulated hernia are similar to colic—constant pain, uneasiness, sweating, and ground pawing.

Treatment is usually surgical with inguinal and scrotal hernias. The unbilical hernia that is common in foals often disappears unaided by the first year of life. If it doesn't, surgery is indicated.

Melanoma

A *melanoma* is a benign (noncancerous) growth found around the tail of gray and white horses. These tumors are rare during the early years, but most often increase in size after fifteen years of age. In rare cases, they can be found on the head, neck, and back.

There is no treatment for melanoma other than surgical means. A

133

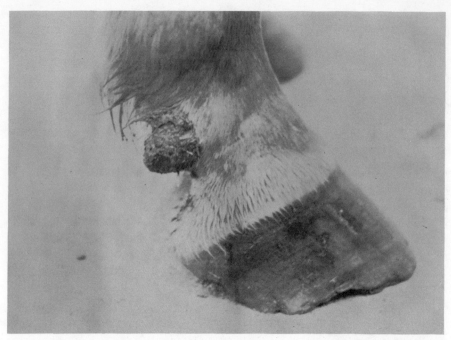

Figure 101. All skin growths and tumors should be examined by a veterinarian to ascertain the difference between a melanoma and a malignant sarcoid, pictured here.

veterinarian should be consulted for diagnosis and future use of a horse with growths (Fig. 101).

Pleurisy

Pleurisy is inflammation of the outer lining of the lungs and chest caused by a bacterial or viral infection. It is generally associated with pneumonia or strangles and inflammation of the sac surrounding the heart.

Because of the inflammation, fluid fills the space between the lining of the chest wall and the outside covering of the lungs. This causes considerable pain to the horse, and his breathing is shallow and rapid.

Treatment for pleurisy is with antibiotic therapy and draining of the fluid to ease breathing difficulties. Pleurisy can be a serious problem—so always get professional veterinary help if you suspect it.

Pneumonia

Pneumonia is an inflammation of lung tissue brought about by fungal, parasitic, bacterial or viral infection, or inhalation of particles or chemicals. It can also be caused mechanically by injury or by fluid being pumped accidentally into the lungs, as with incorrectly adminis-

134

tered worming medicine. Symptoms of pneumonia are an increased rate and depth of breathing, coughing, fever, and a rattling sound or high-pitched tone heard when inhaling, especially, when bronchitis is present with pneumonia.

When bacterial or viral infections are present, single or double pneumonia (one or both lungs) can be diagnosed. The infection, accompanied by difficult breathing and a high temperature, spreads from the bottom of the lung upward. When both lungs are infected, breathing is labored, since there is little oxygen present to sustain life.

When you notice any symptoms of fever, loss of appetite, nasal discharge, and cough, call your veterinarian before the respiratory problem goes too far. Antibiotic treatment is necessary to cure pneumonia.

Purpura Hemorrhagica

Purpura hemorrhagica is a noncontagious, acute disease that flares suddenly and is characterized by purpura swellings or lumps on the stomach, between the legs, or on the tops of the legs. Often the face will develop these cold, painless swellings. They're caused by bleeding into the soft tissues and are characteristic in their square shape and pitting on pressure.

The cause of this disease is unknown, although there is a possibility that it is virally caused, and a sequel to strangles. There is no specific cure and most cases die from blood loss and secondary bacterial infection. Other affected animals respond to injections of antihistamines and corticosteroid drugs, blood transfusions, and rest, particularly when their appetite is good.

Roaring

On either side of the larynx, or voice box, are two flaps that move when the horse breathes. When the nerves that supply the muscles that control these flaps are damaged, the flap ceases to move due to paralysis of the nerve. This results in the flap obstructing the larynx and interfering with the passage of air. When the horse breathes in, there's either a high pitched whistle or a low roaring sound. Due to the reduction of air passing into the lungs, a roarer becomes breathless quickly and cannot be worked strenuously.

Unless both flaps are paralyzed, you cannot tell a roarer unless he's galloped to exertion. The noise will appear at that time.

Whistling and roaring are chronic conditions that will rarely reverse themselves without surgery. The operation is called Hobday's Operation, and when successful, restores the horse to full riding serviceability.

Strangles

   Strangles, or distemper, is a highly infectious bacterial disease common to young horses and those kept in conditions such as a sale barn or lot. When the horse is fatigued by a long trailer ride or poor health, his susceptibility to the disease increases. If the infected animal comes into contact with others, strangles quickly spreads.

   The symptoms are similar to that of a cold. The horse is tired, runs a temperature, has a high pulse, and goes off feed. Internally the mucous membrane of the pharynx becomes inflamed. As the disease progresses, the inflammation causes a pus discharge from the nostrils, a sore throat, painful lymph nodes, and difficulty in swallowing. The lymph nodes may swell until abscesses form and eventually rupture.

   When the abscesses break, the temperature drops and recovery usually follows in two to four weeks. If, however, the infection spreads to tissues surrounding the lymph nodes, abscesses can develop in the liver or kidneys and kill the animal.

   When symptoms of strangles occur, call your veterinarian. The horse should be started on antibotics, isolated, and all equipment used on him disinfected (including your hands).

Sweeny

   The word *sweeny* refers to a wasting (atrophy) of the supraspinatus and infraspinatus shoulder muscles due to disuse or damage to the nerve that supplies the muscles. The must common cause of sweeny, which appears as a noticeable dent or hollowing in the shoulder (Fig. 102), is a blow or severing of the nerve from a kick, injury, or fall.

   Pain and lameness may be absent following the injury, but appear when the muscles begin to atrophy. In some cases, there is often difficulty in extending the shoulder, and the stride shortens on the affected side. As the muscles waste, the shoulder joint is not held as firmly as before and becomes loose, moving away from the body. It's often mistaken for a shoulder dislocation. With advanced sweeny, the leg on the injured side moves in a semicircular course or appears to wing under the body with weight.

   Treatment for this condition, when caused by disuse, is to return the horse to work to rebuild tissue. If sweeny is caused by injury, pasture rest is advocated. Cold compress treatment should be given for twenty-four hours after injury, then followed with hot packs and counterirritants. If the nerve has been severed, recovery to full service is unlikely. Mild cases respond in six to eight weeks, while severe cases with nerve damage may take in excess of three to six months.

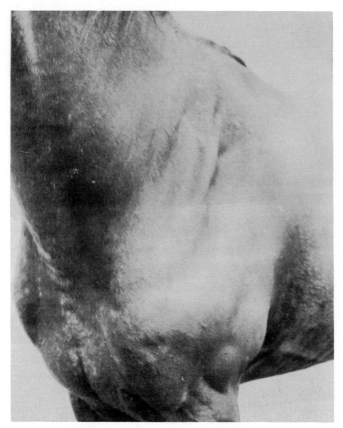

Figure 102. Sweeny of the shoulder caused by falling on a tree stump left in pasture.

Tetanus

Tetanus, also known as lockjaw, is a constant, potential death threat to unimmunized horses. The germ that causes tetanus is common to manure and barnyard soil, and can lie dormant for many years. Some horses do not recover, even with prompt veterinary attention to wounds. Tetanus prevention begins with a yearly vaccination and booster thereafter.

Symptoms of tetanus are an extended muzzle and neck, due to tetanic spasms of the muscles. If the third eyelid moves up over the eye when the chin is elevated, you can be sure the horse has tetanus. With advancing symptoms, breathing becomes labored and opening the mouth is difficult. Eating and drinking becomes impossible.

Treatment without previous antitoxin or toxoid vaccination is usually unsuccessful. A *tetanus antitoxin* gives immediate short-term (two-week) protection. The *tetanus toxoid* stimulates development of active, long-term immunity.

137

7

Pinpointing Lameness and Lamenesses of the Legs

Lameness is not only one of the most common causes of laying up your horse, it is also one of the most frustrating to diagnose as to its source and possible origin. Anywhere between the shoulder and the foot—maybe—and perhaps in the front, but maybe, too, in the back—but where?

If there's a chance that you can supply these answers to your veterinarian when you ask him for help, it'll make his treatment quicker, possibly more accurate, and in many cases, will prevent further damage til he arrives. To learn to pinpoint the trouble site, you'll need to know a few rules of lameness.

1. Have the horse hand-trotted slowly over a hard surface and observe it coming toward and away.

2. If only one leg is lame—in the front—you'll note *the head nodding up on the lame leg and going down when the sound limb hits the ground.* Why? Because the horse uses its head as a counterbalance to keep excessive weight off the injured limb.

3. If lameness is present in both front limbs, nodding of the head will not show. The horse shows symptoms of not moving out as fast or as far as before. If your veterinarian does a nerve block on one limb to take away pain, lameness will then be evident when the unnerved leg hits the ground.

138

4. To differentiate between fore and hindlimb lameness, watch the head. It is slightly thrust forward and down when the lame rear leg hits the ground. Also observe the croup of the rear quarters. With a lower hind leg lameness, the croup of the affected side is usually lowered when the sound leg hits the ground and the opposite hip slightly elevated when the lame leg hits the ground. The opposite is generally the rule in moderate to severe hock joint lameness—the croup of the affected side is carried lower than the normal side.

If you can pinpoint a lame leg, observe the other three and see if there is more than one that is sore. Look at each joint and see if it flexes and extends freely. Watch to see that each stride is full and easily taken. When the horse circles, is lameness accentuated in either direction? When he stands, is one limb pointed, is the toe or heel favored or rested? Does your horse stumble when he moves at either the walk or trot? What about the hindlimbs. Are they coordinated? Does the horse back without shuffling or dragging?

Satisfied that you've zeroed in on the trouble spot(s) and noted physical irregularities, you can proceed to feel, or palpate, the painful region. Note the following:

1. Is there heat in the region? Are there swellings, soft or hard, or obviously painful areas?

2. Palpate the entire leg from the elbow to the coronary band, running your fingers down the length of the tendons at the back of the cannon. Then check the foot. Are there problems such as a nail, cut, thrush, bruise, contracted heel, or crack that might cause pain?

3. If you have hoof testers, apply pressure to the front and quarters of the hoof and see if the animal flinches. Repeat the test on the sound foot to see if a similar reaction occurs.

4. Observe the size and shape of the feet and joints. Are they equal in size, shape, and angle?

5. Are the limbs straight?

6. Flex the joints by picking them up and holding them in a flexed position for several minutes. Then trot the horse straight out and see if there's any noticeable lameness. Was there any evidence of pain when you initially bent the limb?

Even after you've found the seat of pain, you may not be able to localize the site of the lameness. In that case, you'll have to wait until your veterinarian chooses to block the foot nerve(s) with a local anesthetic. Starting with the lowest nerve first, he will work up, trotting the horse to see if lameness leaves.

He will continue working up the leg until various causes are eliminated for the lameness. In many cases, X-rays will be necessary to accurately confirm a diagnosis. Fractures, calcium deposits, and bone bruises show

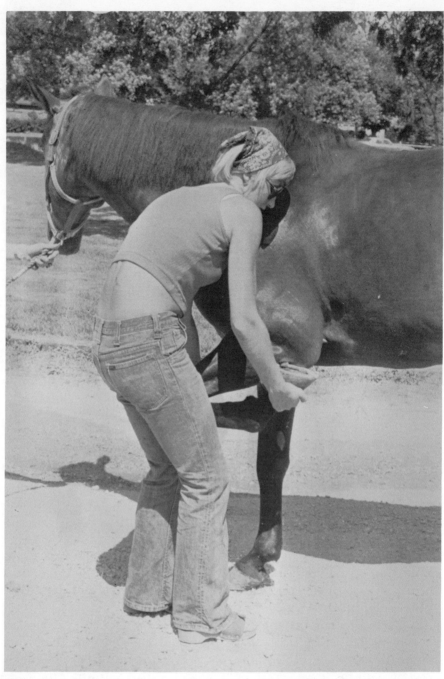

Figure 103. To test for lameness in the front leg, hold up the leg and bend the pastern back for a minute. Before you release the leg, alert the assistant on the lead rope to immediately start the horse moving when you let go.

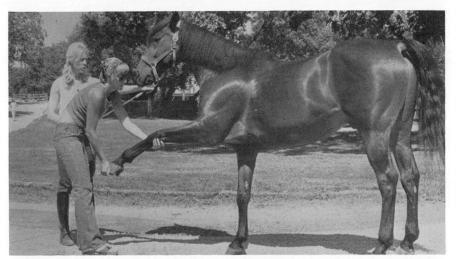

Figure 104. Some shoulder lameness can be detected by holding the foreleg in this position and lifting it gently. If there is a problem in the shoulder, the horse will flinch noticeably.

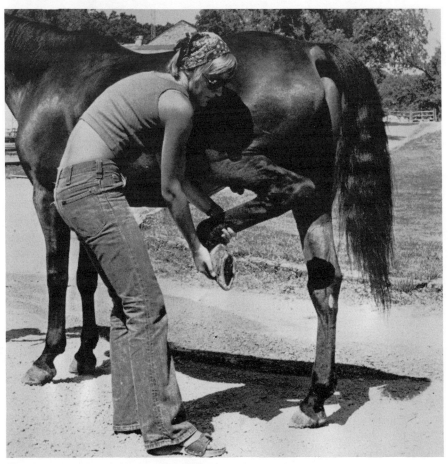

Figure 105. To test for hindleg lameness, lift and hold each leg for a minute and then trot the horse off quickly on a hard surface.

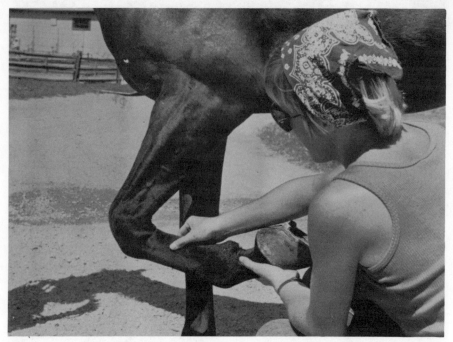

Figure 106. When examining a horse prior to purchase, make sure you feel the tendons for lumps and swelling.

up readily, while injuries to the soft tissue are not visible until calcium deposits develop.

It's helpful to your veterinarian to have an accurate history of the lameness. Note the following:

1. When did the lameness appear? Was it sudden or gradual?

2. Does it become more noticeable after exercise?

3. Is this an old, recurring lameness?

4. What was the horse doing previous to becoming lame? What do you think is the possible cause?

DISEASES OF THE LEG

Arthritis

The word *arthritis* describes inflammation of the hard and soft tissues of a joint. It's of particular importance to you because arthritis interferes with the movement and serviceability of the horse. Arthritis in the equine can be found in three types: acute serous, septic or purulent, and chronic (the most common type seen).

With *acute serous arthritis,* usually only one joint is involved due to an

142

injury or stress. The joint capsule surrounding the joint fills and swells with synovial fluid and blood. It may be hot and sensitive to the touch and cause lameness.

Absolute rest is necessary until the swelling, pain, and lameness disappear. Cold water or ice packs are applied to relieve pain and reduce inflammation. Additional relief is gained when the veterinarian aspirates (withdraws) fluid from the distended joint capsule and injects corticosteroids to reduce inflammation and retard refilling with fluid.

Septior purulent arthritis is characterized by swelling of the joint with pus. It's associated with navel ill in foals or can occur with injuries that penetrate a joint. When bacteria enter the wound, they produce pus, and subsequent inflammation makes this type of arthritis extremely painful. With longstanding cases, or those not treated immediately, there is a chance of bone and cartilage erosion.

Treatment is with systemic antibiotics, given by injection, and topical antibiotic ointments applied daily. Pus within the joint capsule is aspirated and its contents replaced with antibiotics to concentrate aid to the area. During treatment, movement of the joint is very important so that the fibers of the capsule do not thicken and subsequently restrict movement.

Chronic arthritis, also called osteoarthritis, is characterized by a buildup of calcium deposits (exostoses) around the joint, thereby interfering with movement (Fig. 107). These deposits are caused by wear and tear on the joints, early riding, injury, poor conformation, and repeated trauma to the same joint site. Ringbone and bone spavin are examples of chronic arthritis.

Treatment must begin early if stiffness is to be prevented or controlled. Surgical fusion or deposit removal is indicated for chronic arthritis. Following veterinary treatment, rest for several months or more is advocated. Proper nutrition, limited exercise, and elimination of riding stress factors are important in preserving the usefulness of an arthritic horse.

Bowed Tendon

A *bowed tendon* (tendonitis) is a laming disorder caused by injury and subsequent inflammation of one or both of the flexor tendons extending the length of the back of the cannon bone. Turn back to Figure 6 and locate two tendons, the deep and superficial digital flexor tendons. Each is covered with a sheath lubricated by synovial fluid. As explained in the first chapter, this fluid serves to minimize friction between the two tendons. It also produces excess fluid—hence swelling—when there is an injury to the tendons and the sheath.

143

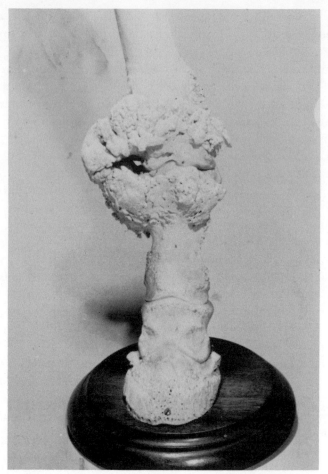

Figure 107. Severe osteoarthritis of the fetlock joint.

A bowed tendon develops primarily in the front leg(s) from over-exertion, training while fatigue is present, fast work through deep going, and hard surfaces and jumping. Improper shoeing that places excess stress on the flexor tendons can also predispose to tendonitis, as can poor conformation and starting work at too early an age. Rupture of the check ligament is often the first sign that the horse has been overstressed and lameness will follow. If the horse is returned to work before the ligament has healed, it, and the tendon, will rupture further.

When the horse is overstressed, the tendon fibers rupture, and bleeding and swelling quickly follow. The horse's weight is transferred to the toe, so as to ease pressure on the tendon(s). Many horses, not allowed enough rest to heal, will bow the same tendon repeatedly. This chronic bowing causes a shortening and thickening of the tendon.

144

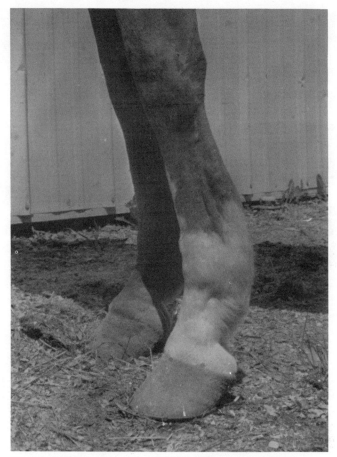
Figure 108. An old, set bowed tendon in a jumper.

Avoiding a chronic case of tendonitis depends heavily on how quickly the horse is treated and how long he's laid up. Even after healing, a bowed tendon will never be as strong as preinjury, and care must be taken not to stress the part.

Initial treatment is with cold packs to reduce swelling and inflammation. Many veterinarians prefer to immobilize the leg with a cast for six to eight weeks, while others treat the injury with drugs and stall rest for several weeks. The leg must be supported with bandages for approximately four weeks after removal of the cast, when this treatment method is used, followed by twelve months rest before exercise is resumed.

Bucked Shins
Bucked shins is an inflammation or tearing of the periosteum of the

145

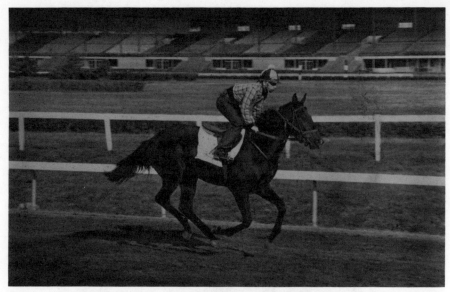

Figure 109. Bowed tendons are common in race horses, since their extreme youth and stressful occupation ruptures tendons.

cannon bone(s) of the front leg(s). It is less frequently seen in the hind. Sore shins is a problem common to young race horses, or those immature horses subject to hard training and severe stress. In horses older than three years of age, injury can cause bucked shins.

When the periosteum, or membranous covering of the cannon bone, is torn from the front surface of the bone, bleeding and subsequent swelling occur. In severe cases, fracture of the cannon also accompanies the tearing. If you palpate the area, you'll find it warm and painful. Lameness is sometimes evident. When a horse is exercised after this injury, his stride becomes noticeably shorter and the severity of lameness increases.

Treatment for bucked shins begins with complete rest and withdrawal from all exercise. Cold packs and bandages will reduce inflammation, along with antiinflammatory drugs. Note that these drugs also alleviate pain symptoms, so lameness usually disappears. Do not work your horse at this time, since exercise would cause further damage to the site and result in thickening of the anterior surface of the leg(s).

Capped Hock and Capped Elbow
On the point of the hock and at the point of the elbow is a bursa that fills with excess synovial fluid when injured. Trauma occurs from lying on hard floors, riding the trailer tailgate, falling, being kicked, or from long periods of illness forcing recumbency.

Lameness is infrequent with these synovial distensions, regardless of the size of the swellings.

If treated with cold water or cold packs during their early stages, plus aspiration and corticosteroid injections, the size may be reduced. Surgical removal may be advocated for those bursa which are encapsulated or have abscesses (Fig. 110). To further prevent irritation of the capped hock or capped elbow, you can bandage the hock and use a shoeboil roll to prevent the hind shoe from hitting the elbow (Fig. 111).

Carpitis

The term *carpitis* (carpus-knee, itis-inflammation) is also called big knee, sore knee, and popped knee (Fig. 112). It is common to young horses in racing training, and in hunters and jumpers that have hit and injured their knees. In cases of longstanding knee banging in the stall, sore knees may also develop. Poor conformation of the forelegs may predispose a horse to carpitis.

Inflammation of the area brings on lameness and swelling. In chronic cases, bony growth may appear. Fracture of one or more of the small carpal bones may be present, necessitating withdrawal from work.

Treatment consists of rest and withdrawal of fluid from the knee. Injection of a corticosteroid will help relieve pain. In the case of long-standing carpitis, degenerative changes in the bone usually indicate

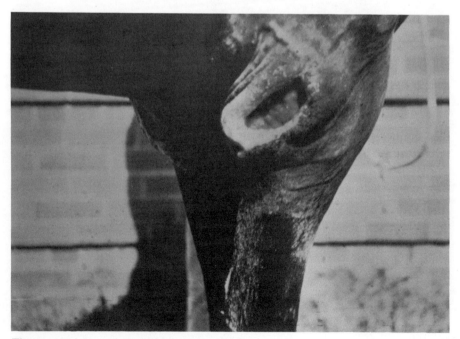

Figure 110. An ulcerated shoe boil.

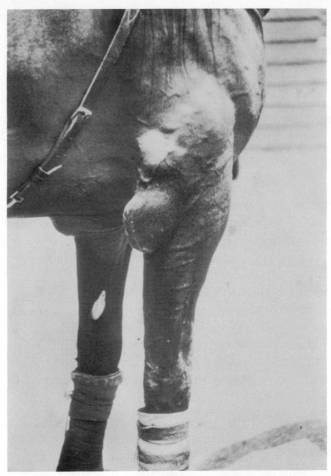

Figure 111. A severe case of shoe boils caused from striking the point of the elbow with the rear foot.

that the horse will not be fully sound in the future and should be withdrawn from its present, stressful work.

Curb

Approximately six inches below the point of the hock, at the back of the upper end of the cannon bone, is the site for development of *curb*. Due to poor conformation in the hock area, injury, stress (Fig. 113), or sprain, the plantar ligament thickens or bows. A curb is easily seen when viewing the horse from the side. It is characterized by lameness in the beginning stages of development, along with an elevated heel and weighted toe when at rest.

Treatment with cold packs and rest is helpful during the first stages of curb development to reduce inflammation. When the curb is "set,"

148

point-firing over the enlarged ligament may be indicated, along with prolonged rest. A gradual return to exercise is advisable.

Osselets

The word *osselets* is a term loosely referring to any enlargement of the fetlocks. The condition causing the enlargement is usually repeated injury due to severe training while young, as in race horses. With strain and stress, the fetlock joint and the fibrous joint capsule surrounding it become inflamed.

During its acute first stage, pain and lameness are evident, and the horse shortens its stride and develops a choppy gait. Any palpation and flexion of the joint produces pain. The joint is warm, painful, and enlarged over the front and sides of the joint (Fig. 114).

If X rays reveal no buildup of new bone, the condition is termed

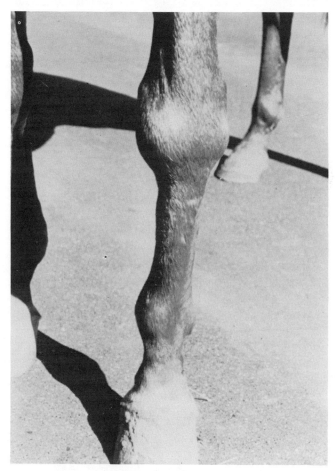

Figure 112. Big knee in an advanced stage.

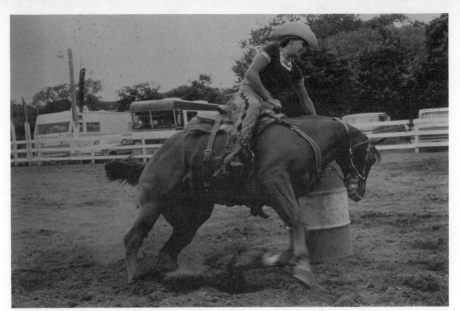

Figure 113. Every muscle of this barrel horse shows the strain of its profession and is an indication of the stress put on its joints.

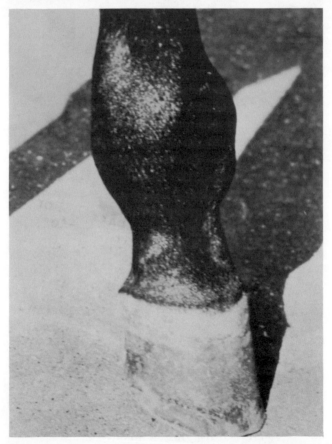

Figure 114. Osteoarthritis, or osselets, of the fetlock joint.

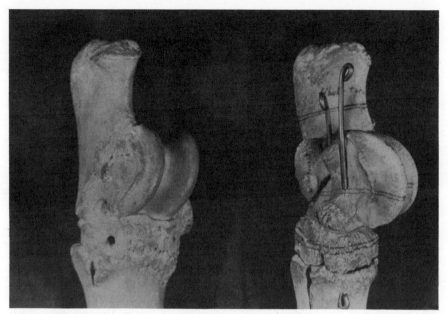

Figure 115. Normal hock on right, bone spavin on left.

green osselets. In later stages, bone demineralization and osteoarthritic lesions are evident. The terminal stage is characterized by calcium buildup and permanent enlargement of the ankle.

All training should be suspended and the horse rested at the first sign of osselets. Cold packs and antiinflammatory drugs are indicated. Additional treatment measures include poulticing until inflammation subsides. A long rest is critical, since the joint capsule can be seriously damaged and torn with continued work. Once inflammation has subsided, and sufficient rest given, prognosis for future serviceability is good.

Spavin

A *spavin* is a condition of the hock joint, or its surrounding capsule, which may result in lameness. There are two main types of spavin, bog and bone.

Bog spavin is a firm swelling of the hock joint occurring over the front inside surface of the hock, or on either side of the hock, below the point of the hock (Fig. 115). The swellings are the result of increased synovial fluid production by the tibia-tarsal joint capsule, and are largely caused by the stress of faulty hock conformation. Nutritional deficiencies or excesses, injuries, and bacterial or viral infections may also contribute to formation of bog spavin.

Unless complicated by arthritis or a fracture within the hock area, lameness is not usually present. The swellings do not often interfere with the serviceability of the horse, but do cause blemishes that render the horse unfit for showing in some classes.

Treatment to reduce swelling consists of aspirating the fluid within the joint capsule and injecting it with corticosteroids. This method may produce only temporary results, since recurrence of swelling is commonplace, especially with poorly conformed horses. Blisters and linaments generally yield poor, long-term results in reducing the swellings. Manual massage several times daily, in addition to pressure bandages, may be helpful in reducing swelling.

A *bone spavin* begins with an inflamed bone or periosteum in the small tarsal joints of the hock. This is followed by progressive degeneration of the bone, a form of osteoarthritis. The final outcome, in most cases, is calcium buildup, bone erosion, and stiffening of the joint (ankylosis).

Lameness is present, and the horse tends to drag its toe and shorten the stride. Hock action is stiff, and when standing, the heel is raised. Some horses work out of lameness with exercise and become lame after resting. If the bone lesion is within the moving surfaces of the bones, lameness doesn't disappear, since exercise irritates the condition. In some horses the pain may be so severe that if the animal is made to put weight on the hock after standing in a trailer or after arising from the ground, you'll note the leg being jerked up quickly. While pain and lameness are most severe in the initial acute stages, they tend to disappear once ankylosis of the small tarsal joints is complete.

The causes for bone spavin are the same as bog spavin: poor conformation, nutritional excesses or deficiencies, injury, and stress and overwork. Horses used in work that demands excess wear and tear on the hindlimbs, such as reining work and jumping (Fig. 116), are more prone to having spavins than other work classifications.

In treating bone spavin, X rays are taken to note bone changes in the hock. Then the veterinarian chooses from several methods of treatment. Some favor point-firing to hasten ankylosis, others favor arthrodesis— the stiffening of the joint by surgical means. Some horses respond well to corrective shoeing with heel raising and rolled-toed shoes. Surgical separation of calcium buildups may reduce pain if they rub a tendon. Another method is to remove a portion of the cunean tendon (jack cord) in the hock to eliminate pain.

With proper treatment, a good percentage of affected horses return to service. The prognosis for this depends on the site of the spavin, the type of spavin, and the length of time the horse can be rested.

Splints

On either side of the horse's cannon bone are two rudimentary and

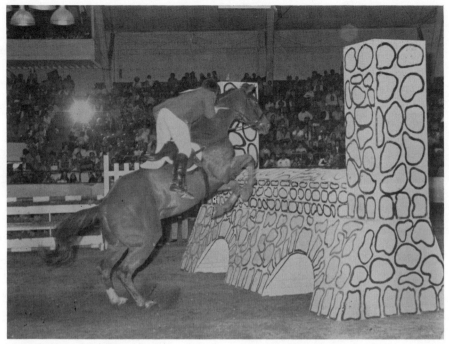

Figure 116. Jumping puts tremendous strain on the hocks and pasterns. Look at the effort the hindquarters is making to launch the horse over the jump.

slender splint bones (Fig. 117). They're held to the cannon bone by ligaments that allow limited up and down movement as the horse puts weight on the leg. If the horse is asked to overexert—especially when immature—or receives a kick, suffers from a nutritional imbalance or faulty conformation, a splint can occur.

What happens is the ligament binding the splint bone tears and the bone moves more than it should. This irritates the cannon bone and further damages the ligament. Acute pain and swelling appear and become more marked when the horse is worked. At first, there may be no enlargement of the area, but eventually, new bone is laid down and in many cases, the splint bone becomes ankylosed to the cannon bone. When this occurs—and after the bone inflammation subsides—the splint is no longer painful to the horse.

Treatment for splint begins with X rays to differentiate between simple splint and a fractured splint bone. If the end of the splint bone is fractured, surgical removal of the fragment is indicated. In the normal splint reaction, rest from training and massaging of the splint enlargement may be the only treatment needed.

You can do a lot to prevent splints by using boots designed to protect the inside cannon area while training a young horse. Many splints occur

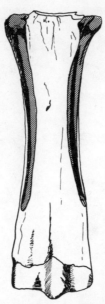

Figure 117. Rear view of the cannon bone with splint bone in normal position.

when the animal hits itself with the opposite limb. It's also a wise precaution to put boots on when longeing a horse, regardless of age.

Stringhalt

Stringhalt refers to a condition characterized by a hyperflexed spasm of one or both rear legs during movement. It can affect any breed, at any age, but its cause is not known. Autopsies of afflicted horses have revealed lesions and degeneration of the spinal cord and specific nerves, in some cases—possibly a cause of the disease.

Flexion of the joints ranges from mild to severe, and intermittent to continuous. The condition is most evident when the horse is backed or sharply pivoted. Frequently, other ailments such as thrush, mange, weed allergy, or dermatitis of the ankle or pastern will cause the horse to lift its feet sharply, so a prompt veterinary diagnosis is indicated before suspecting stringhalt.

Treatment for stringhalt is most successful with surgical resection of part of an extensor tendon in the afflicted leg. Even after healing, the horse may not return to serviceability. This disease is considered an *unsoundness*, even though it may not hinder the horse's suitability for its job.

Thoroughpin

Thoroughpin refers to an in or outside (or both) swelling in front of

154

the point of the hock, caused when the tendon sheath of the deep flexor tendon at the hock fills with synovial fluid. This filling is due to faulty hock conformation, injury, or overwork. With longstanding cases, the swelling may also extend to the outside surface of the hock.

Lameness is not usually evident, and treatment should be confined to fluid aspiration and rest. The primary objective in the initial stage is to reduce swelling so the enlargement is not permanent. If the horse will tolerate pressure bandages on the hock, these will help reduce swelling. Exercise should be resumed slowly.

Tying-Up

Tying-up, Monday morning disease, or azoturia, is usually seen in regularly worked horses that have been idle for a day or two fully fed. On the day following rest on full feed, the horse shows symptoms of severe muscle cramping, hanging back, and hindlimb lameness. If not stopped immediately, he will fall and may not be able to rise. Sweating and blowing also accompany this disease.

When stiffness occurs after a day of rest, contact your veterinarian. Massage the hindlegs and cut down on feed. Prevention consists of lowering feed while off work and keeping exercise constant. When ill, give laxative feeds.

Windpuffs

At the back of the fetlock joint are tendons, surrounded by a digital

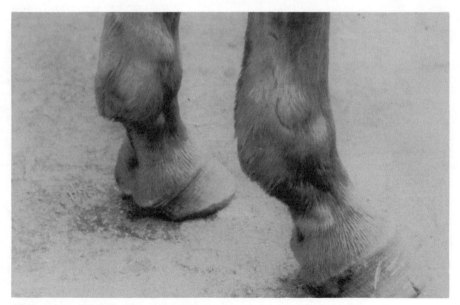

Figure 118. Windpuffs on both forelegs of a jumper.

155

sheath that produces excess synovial fluid when inflamed (Fig. 118). The excess fluid causes swelling, (visible on either side of the tendon) which can occur in both fore and hind fetlocks. This digital sheath distention is called a *windpuff* or *windgall*. Generally, windpuffs are indications that the horse has been overstressed, thus causing tearing of the tendon or tendon sheath fibers. If the horse is not lame from them, the swellings are considered a blemish, rather than unsoundness.

Treatment for the condition in its inflammatory stage is aspiration of fluid and injection of antiinflammatory drugs into the site. As with most synovial distentions, the area refills in time and remains filled, usually presenting no problem to the horse's serviceability.

8

Problems of the Foot

Regardless of how clean you keep your horse's feet and how often you attend to trimming and shoeing, the stresses on those four small parts of the horse's total anatomy take their toll now and then. It's impossible to guard against injury from accidental causes, injury due to faulty conformation, and diseases of the foot to any great degree. Familiarity with some of the common problems of the foot will, however, enable you to spot many conditions before they worsen and get immediate attention for the problem.

Buttress Foot

Buttress foot, or pyramidal disease, occurs at the top front surface of the coffin bone (third phalanx) in the area of the extensor or pyramidal process (Fig. 119). When this process is fractured or hit with force, inflammation of the periosteum and bone begins. Usually the common digital extensor tendon, which inserts on the extensor process, is also torn, thereby causing extreme pain and lameness.

Heat and swelling are evident at the coronary band directly over the process. As the disease progresses, this area will bulge and assume a boxy, buttresslike appearance. In many cases, the foot will contract, leading to secondary foot complications.

X rays are necessary to diagnose the presence of a fracture. If chips are present, surgical removal is recommended. In most cases of buttress foot the prognosis is poor. The disease usually develops into arthritis of the coffin joint with resulting irritation and chronic lameness.

157

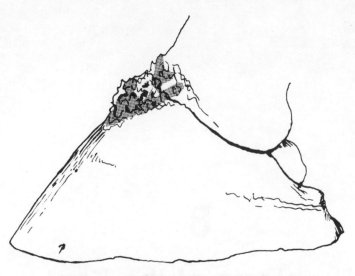

Figure 119. Buttress foot or pyramidal disease.

Contracted Heels

Contracted heels is a condition characterized by a narrowing of the heel area (Fig. 120), and sometimes the entire foot. It is mostly seen in one or both front feet and is usually the result of lack of normal expansion of the foot. This can be due to many causes, from dry hooves and lack of exercise to chronic, low-grade pain in the limb, especially in the heel area of the foot. Contracted heels can also result from improper shoeing, shoes left on too long, very long feet, or as the result of a disease (thereby making it a secondary complication).

Lameness may be evident at fast and hard work, and be accompanied by a shortening of stride. Heat around the heels and sides of the foot may also be present. These symptoms are usually caused by the lesion or disease leading to contracted heels.

Treatment begins with a thorough examination of the feet by a veterinarian to treat both primary and secondary problems. The aim is to restore frog pressure through corrective trimming to allow proper expansion of the foot. When treating this condition, it's very important to apply a hoof dressing daily to keep the foot soft. A pliable hoof will allow expansion without cracking. Quite often, a bar shoe is used to put pressure on the frog and aid it in pushing out the quarters of the hoof. Recovery may take up to a year, since it involves periodic shoeing along with curing the original cause of contracted heels.

Corns and Bruised Sole

When the sole of the foot, between the wall and the bar, is bruised,

158

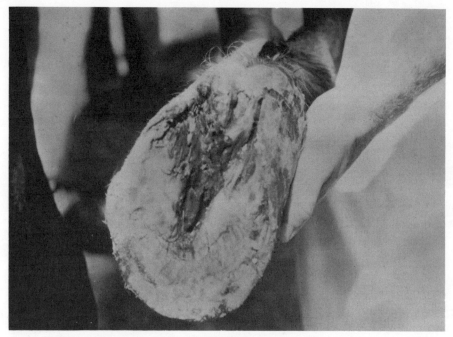

Figure 120. Contracted heels and atrophied frog.

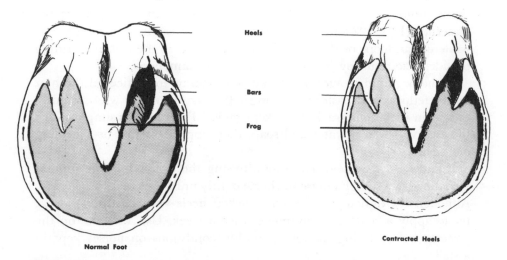

Heels

Bars

Frog

Normal Foot

Contracted Heels

Figure 121. The normal foot on the left shows a well-formed, wide sole at the quarters and a broad expanse of heel. The frog is wide enough to permit ground contact and expansion of the foot. The contracted foot on the right shows an obvious lack of breadth at the heel area and frog, thereby limiting the expansion of the foot. Notice, too, that the sole is somewhat narrower than the healthy foot.

159

a lesion known as a *corn* develops. Lameness is usually the first indication of the presence of a corn. Upon closer inspection, you will see a red or yellowish-red discoloration that is sensitive to tapping or pressure.

Treatment starts with finding the cause. If the corn was the result of a bad shoeing or shoes long overdue to be changed, alert your farrier and veterinarian. The next step is to relieve pressure and pain from the corn site by cutting out bruised tissue and putting on a corrective shoe.

If the corn is infected, it is usually drained with a surgical opening in the sole. This relieves internal pressure and pain on the foot. Soaking the foot and keeping the horse in a clean stall is necessary to prevent further bacterial complications.

A *bruised sole* is a term that refers to a bruise on the front or volar aspect of the sole. The cause may result from improper shoeing of animals with a dropped sole or flat feet, but may also occur from stepping on stones or other sharp objects.

A bruised sole resembles the corn in color, but tends to become infected more quickly and spread under the horn of the sole. Immediate attention to the feet is necessary to relieve pressure and pain. The shoes are removed and the sole pared, poulticed, and the horse confined to a stall for a week or more.

Cracked Heels

The term *cracked heels* would be more anatomically specific if worded *cracked pasterns*, since the irritation is actually on the rear side of the pastern(s) (Figs. 122 and 123). This condition is usually found on horses wintered outdoors, or those left with mud caked to the feet after riding outside. The resulting irritation may lead to lameness.

In the beginning stages, scabs and skin flaking are noticed if the hair on the fetlocks and pastern is clipped. Just like your dry winter hands, these skin irritations crack if not kept moist. Treatment is simple: wash the area with warm water and soap, then apply Vaseline or a healing ointment.

If lameness is evident, continue dressing the area while the animal is confined to a stall. Exercise the horse lightly until the cracks are healed. Although it's difficult to prevent cracked heels with pastured horses, try to apply a coating of ointment twice a week. Use Vaseline on the pasterns before riding in wet or muddy conditions on horses kept in a stall.

Cracked Hooves

Cracks in the hoof wall result from improper foot care, thin walls, no shoes, neglect, drying out from lack of moisture or hoof dressing, and work on hard surfaces.

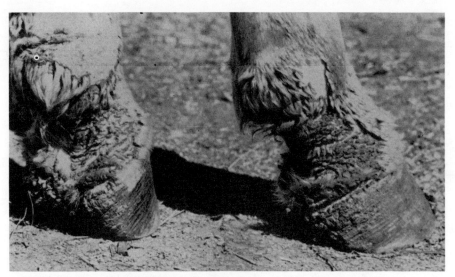
Figure 122. Cracked heels before treatment.

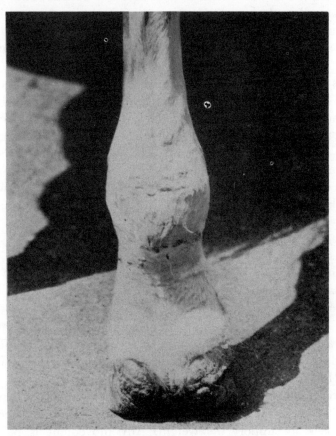
Figure 123. The same pasterns one week after treatment.

Expert corrective shoeing is necessary to prevent the cracks from extending upward into the coronary band or penetrating into the sensitive internal hoof structures. With proper care, the toe and quarter cracks disappear in time through normal horn growth.

Foot Abscess

When a horse steps on a nail, has one accidentally driven into the sensitive internal hoof during shoeing, or has a sharp object penetrate the foot, infection leads to pus formation (suppuration).

Lameness is usually immediately evident if the foreign object damages the sensitive tissues. In most cases, though, lameness appears up to a week after penetration. It takes about this much time for the bacteria on the foreign object to produce enough pus to build up painful pressure within the foot.

If you tap the hoof wall or sole with a hammer, or squeeze it with hoof testers, pain is quite evident. Treatment consists of locating the penetration site—which has closed over with small objects—and opening it enough to allow draining and removal of the object.

The more time that elapses before the object is removed and the wound attended to, the more severe the infection and pain. This is because the pus, which is under considerable pressure within the small confines of the foot, moves into the area between the sensitive laminae and the sole, or between the wall and the laminae. It may then break open and drain at the coronary band.

Once the foot has been drained and flushed with an antibiotic solution, tincture of iodine should be instilled and a cotton plug placed in the drainage hole in the sole. If the hole is large, the foot may have to be bandaged for protection until it is healed, usually one to two weeks. If your horse is not on a tetanus toxoid program, your veterinarian will give a tetanus antitoxin shot.

Laminitis

Laminitis means inflammation of the sensitive laminae of the feet, particularly the front ones. As with most diseases, this one can be a one-time, acute attack, or a chronic one.

With *acute laminitis*, the onset of pain, foot heat, temperature rise, and elevation in pulse and respiration are sudden. If only the front feet are involved, the horse will try supporting his weight on the hindquarters (Fig. 124). This gives him a characteristic look of front feet stretched out in front and rear legs placed far up under the body. When the rear legs are affected, the rear limbs are under the body and the forelegs placed back to support the weight. Any movement is painful and resisted by the horse.

162

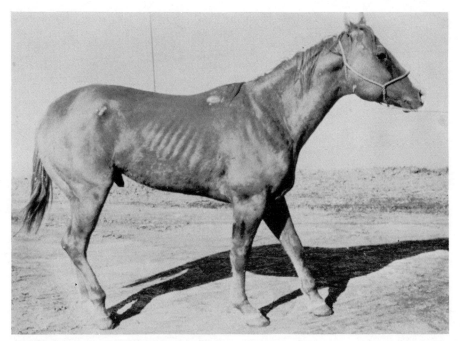

Figure 124. Typical position of a horse with laminitis.

Chronic laminitis is seen after the acute phase has passed and the horse seemingly recovered. Lameness may be mild to severe, with intermittent attacks. Horses are most likely to become chronic if the initial attack was severe and accompanied by downward rotation of the coffin bone inside the hoof.

Why does the coffin bone change its position? When the sensitive laminae become inflamed, serum infiltrates the space between the union of the insensitive and sensitive laminae. This gap created between an otherwise firm union causes a lowering of the front portion of the coffin bone toward the sole. The strong pull of the deep flexor tendon at the back of the bone, plus the horse's weight, assist in pulling the lamina away from the horny wall.

The causes of laminitis include drinking cold water when hot, insufficient cooling after work, overeating grain, hard work on hard surfaces, hard work when out of condition, and numerous other causes. The disease may occur after the horse has been overly purged with a medicine to stimulate bowel movements, or after a respiratory disease or foaling.

Treatment consists of first finding the cause of the laminitis and dealing with it. If overeating, for example, is the cause, then mineral oil may be given to quickly remove the toxins within the body before they're absorbed. Prompt veterinary treatment aims at arresting the disease before the coffin bone rotates and causes a dropped sole.

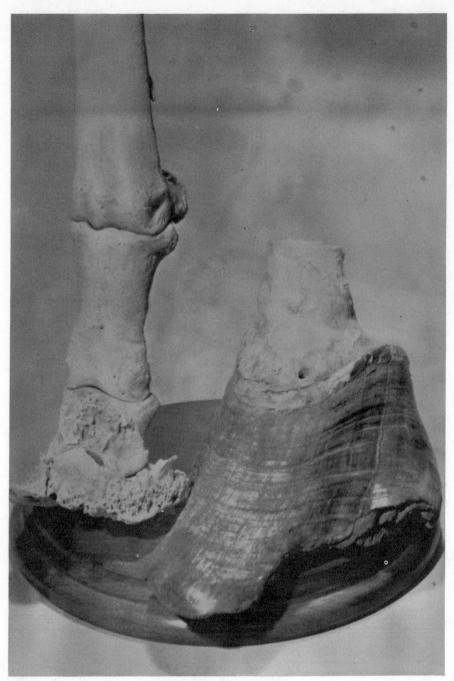

Figure 125. An advanced case of founder.

Cold packs are used by some veterinarians, along with treatment to reduce inflammation. Hot packs are advocated as beneficial by other veterinarians. If you're in doubt as to which method to use until your veterinarian arrives, use cold packs or running water and do not give any drugs or drenches. *The cause of the disease requires a different treatment in each case, and self-diagnosis and treatment may severely complicate the problem.*

With chronic laminitis, treatment consists of restoring the animal to serviceability by realigning the pedal bone. Corrective shoeing is necessary for this. The object is to lower the heels, remove excess toe, and protect the sole from ground contact. Pads, a bar shoe, or acrylic plastic correction are used to achieve realigning. Subsequent care and trimming, plus a low-calorie, high-protein diet are important in preventing chronic attacks.

In cases where the pedal bone has penetrated the sole (Fig. 126), chances for recovery are very doubtful.

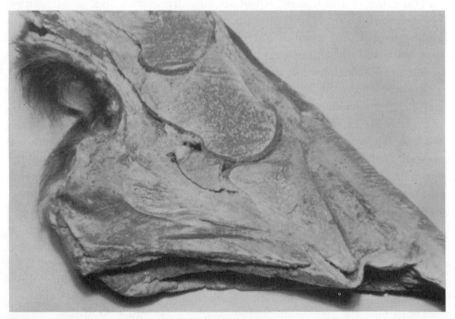

Figure 126. Cross-section of a severely foundered hoof. Note that the coffin bone has rotated down and has dropped the sole.

Navicular Disease

Navicular disease describes a number of degenerative changes in the navicular bone (distal sesamoid) located at the back of the coffin joint (Fig. 127). The disease is a chronic inflammation of this bone and inflammation of the navicular bursa.

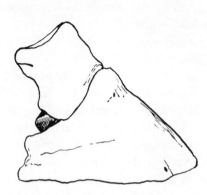

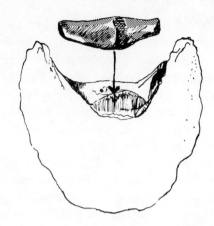

Side View of Foot with Navicular Bone in Position at the Back

Sole of Coffin Bone with Navicular Bone Above Its Normal Position

Figure 127. The navicular bone.

The cause of the disease is not specifically known, but is attributed to hard work on hard surfaces, jumping, poor conformation such as upright pasterns and a small narrow foot, defective shoeing, nutritional and hormonal imbalances, and injury to the navicular area. The disease is most common between the ages of six to nine years.

In some cases, the articular cartilage of the navicular bone becomes irritated by excessive rubbing against the deep flexor tendon running over it. This is the result of concussion and movement while being worked. If a horse has a small, narrow foot, or shrunken frog, the foot has to cope with more concussion than a normally shaped foot. When the bursa becomes traumatized, excess blood is present and degeneration of the bone begins.

In the initial stages of navicular disease, the horse will not extend as before and may stumble. Later, more severe lameness is observed. It may disappear with exercise at first, but later will become persistent and noticeable with hard work. Pointing of the affected foot (Fig. 128), or shuffling from one painful foot to the other—when both are diseased—is characteristic.

Treatment for navicular disease consists of relieving inflammation and pain and shoeing correctly. The heel of the foot is left long, and the toe shortened to raise the angle of the foot. If rest and conservative treatment do not improve the condition, surgery is necessary to relieve pain. The operation is called a *posterior digital* (heel) *neurectomy*. It is performed in both feet and eliminates pain because the two posterior digital nerves at the back of each pastern are severed. This leaves sensation in the front of the foot and the skin, but deadens feeling in the heel area of each foot.

166

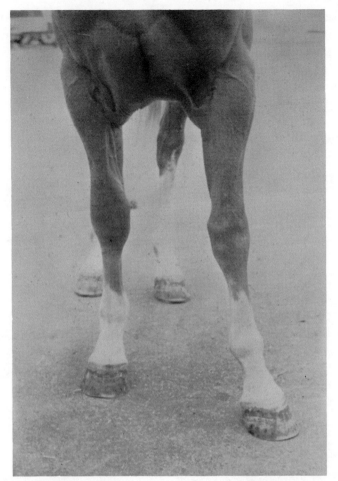

Figure 128. Typical pointing attitude of a navicular diseased horse.

It's important in a denerved horse to check the front feet carefully after each ride. If a nail is picked up, or any area bruised or injured in the heel area, the horse will not feel it. Pads are usually advocated for the front shoes as insurance against stone bruises.

Quittor

Quittor refers to a pus-producing inflammation and tissue death (necrosis) of a lateral cartilage. The pus forms a sinus tract from the cartilage to the coronary band region where it ruptures and drains. Initial indications of a problem are lameness, accompanied by a painful swelling over the inside or outside lateral cartilage. Once the swelling ruptures, lameness subsides as pressure is relieved.

Quittor is caused by a blow or cut to the lateral cartilage. Puncture wounds of the sole may also cause cartilage necrosis. Conformation problems that produce an interfering gait and constant hitting of the cartilage area are also responsible for the condition.

To decide on the method of treatment, the veterinarian has to determine the extent of damage to the nearby joint capsule. In most cases, medical treatment with drugs is unsuccessful, and removal of the diseased cartilage is mandatory. When quittor is treated early in its development, the majority of patients return to serviceability.

Ringbone

The word *ringbone* is a general term used to indicate enlargement of the pastern area (Fig. 129 and 130). The bones involved are the first and second phalanges and the joints between the first and second phalanges (pastern joint), and the second and third phalanges (coffin joint).

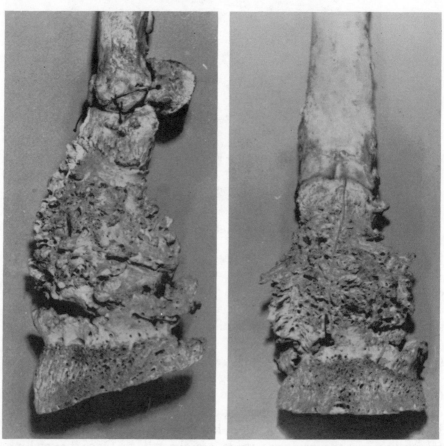

Figures 129 and 130. Two views of a severe case of ringbone involving the pastern and coffin joints. Note the amount of calcium buildup on the extensor process of the coffin bone in Figure 129.

168

Ringbone is usually classified in two ways, somewhat confusing, but definitive:
1. *non-articular*—not involving the pastern or coffin joint
   articular—involving the pastern or coffin joint
2. *high ringbone*—involving the pastern joint
   low ringbone—involving the coffin joint

Ringbone is most common in the front limbs and is characterized by acute to slowly developing lameness, accompanied by swelling of the affected joint. Lameness is the result of inflammation of the periosteum, or osteoarthritis of the joint. It flares up or persists in chronic cases due to bone growth and tissue irritation. As the disease progresses, the affected joint may ankylose. The horse may or may not be pain-free and serviceable when this happens.

Treatment for acute cases begins with total rest and no work. If the joint is not involved, or if bone growth has not started in a joint, cold and astringent applications are recommended.

Seedy Toe

Seedy toe is a separation of the insensitive hoof wall from the sensitive laminae, or quick, due to degeneration of the horn substance. This condition can result from using tight-fitting toe clips, as a sequel to chronic laminitis, because of a crack between the wall and sole, or due to neglect.

Once the wall begins to separate from the laminae, debris and foreign objects pack into the cavity. If an abscess forms, the infection can lead to further foot complications and bone involvement. Seedy toe lameness may be absent or severe, depending upon the extent of the infection.

Treatment consists of removing debris and cutting out diseased tissue. The cavity is then packed with tar and oakum, or antibiotic soaked cotton, and the horse fitted with a shoe to cover the cavity.

Sidebones

When the normally soft, elastic lateral cartilages on either side of the coffin bone harden, or ossify, the condition is called *sidebones* (Fig. 131). It is commonly seen in the front feet of horses worked at fast speeds on hard ground, in hunters and jumpers, as the result of a blow to that area of the foot, and in poorly conformed horses.

Lameness may be present in the acute ossifying stage, but when all inflammation has subsided, sidebones are not a cause of lameness. There is no surgical treatment indicated if lameness is not evident, but corrective shoeing is advised to prevent or aid a contracted foot.

169

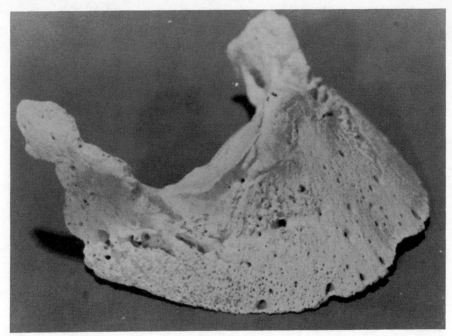

Figure 131. An advanced case of sidebones.

Thrush

   Thrush is a bacterial or fungus-caused infection of the frog that causes degeneration of the horn. It starts in the grooves on either side of the frog due to dirty, wet, urine-soaked stall bedding, and unpicked feet. When left untreated, the infection causes a foul odor acccompanied by a dark discharge.

   As the condition progresses, the grooves and the frog become moist, and sensitivity to probing with the hoof pick is noticeable. In severe cases, thrush gets into the sensitive internal hoof tissues and can cause lameness.

   Treatment in mild cases consists of keeping the stall clean and picking the feet daily. Then use a thrush preparation such as copper naphthenate (available commercially). With more severe cases, the diseased tissue should be trimmed out and the frog grooves packed with gauze and medication obtained from your veterinarian or farrier.

9

Breeding and Foaling

Large-scale breeding and raising of horses are primarily professional specialties, but backyard operations, on a much smaller scale, can be successful and rewarding. A basic knowledge of breeding and foaling, however, is essential and makes your endeavor much more interesting.

Let's start with the *mare*, since most owners find it easier to keep a mare in their yard or stable than a stallion. Months ahead of the breeding date you should be getting her in condition with plenty of exercise and a balanced diet with vitamin and mineral supplementation. She should have her reproductive organs checked and a culture taken to be sure there's no infection present.

If she's never been bred before, the *maiden mare* needs her reproductive organs examined to ascertain if her genital tract is infantile, if the uterus is correctly placed, and if there is a hymen or vaginal septum present that could be torn during breeding (Fig. 132).

A *barren mare* should also be examined to see why she has not conceived in the past before you breed her or continue to breed her without results.

You should consider your mare's age before you consider breeding her. If she's under five years of age, she's still growing and not fully developed herself. Although many mares are bred at age two and three, the longer you wait, the less chance you'll have with her growth being negatively affected by the demands of the foal. With a healthy, though aged mare, regardless of whether she's maiden, chances are good she'll conceive, even into her twenties.

171

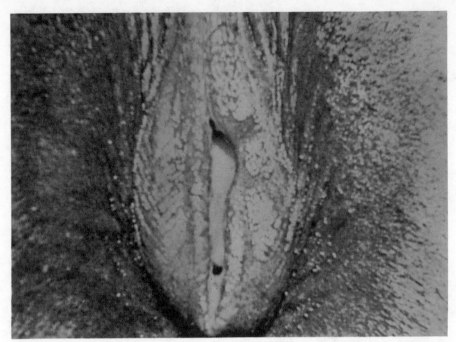

Figure 132. A torn vulva or internal laceration and bruises can often be prevented by having a maiden mare examined before attempting to breed her.

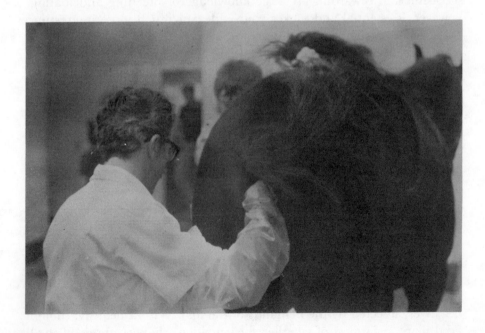

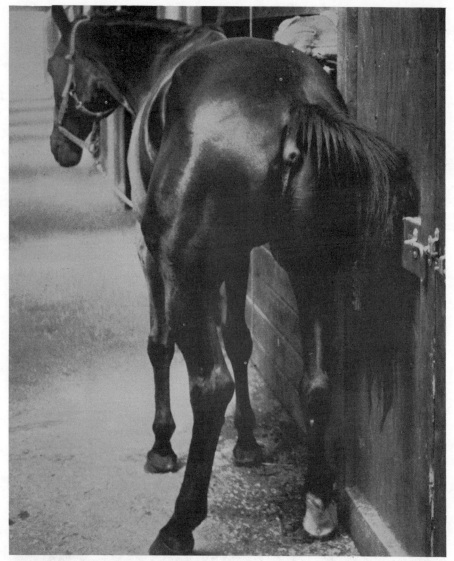

Figure 133. Mare in heat showing typical characteristics of crouched position, lifted tail, and dribbling urine.

The Heat Period

How do you know when your mare shows *heat*? In most mares there are definite signs exhibited at the time the egg is shed from the ovary and she's willing to accept a stallion. The majority of mares crouch down and "present" themselves around geldings, stallions, and sometimes, mares. They also contract, or "wink" their vulva, and spray urine when in heat (Fig. 133).

Heat periods may run in very regular cycles, or be so irregular it's hard to chart them. Some mares have a cycle every twenty-one days with heat lasting four to seven days. Others go through only three cycles per year, and still more exhibit no noticeable signs, but are able to conceive without difficulty. Your veterinarian will be able to help you recognize and chart your mare's heat period after he examines her. Many mares will need to be teased by a stallion one or two months before being bred to bring them into noticeable heat for charting purposes.

Since the mare stays in receptive heat for only three to five days, a veterinarian should check the mare regularly to see if the egg has ruptured its follicle in the ovary. If the stallion services the mare too long before, or too long after ovulation, conception will not take place. Most breeders have their stallion cover the mare every other day to ensure that the sperm—which lives thirty-six to forty-eight hours—will have a chance to unite with the egg. If conception does take place, you'll know after forty to sixty days with a rectal examination or blood test.

When To Breed

The *gestation time*, from conception to birth, is from ten to twelve months, with eleven months being the average. Since the warm spring months are ideal for the foaling date, plan to breed eleven months before the first warm month of spring.

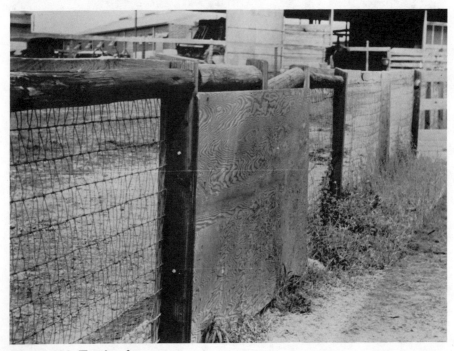

Figure 134. Teasing bar.

Foaling outside and having access to good pasture and sun are important for a healthy foal. While many youngsters start their lives in winter (Fig. 135), some health problems—such as colds—can be avoided by giving the foal a spring birthdate.

Should you plan to register the foal, ask about the breed registry date. If they count the age of the horse from January 1, have the foal born as early in the year as possible to give maximum size for his predated birthday.

Picking the Stallion

One of the most important aspects of breeding is the choice of the *sire*. Pick a stallion with good conformation and disposition. If your mare has a glaring conformation fault—such as cow hocks—look for a stallion with strong hindleg quality. If you want to breed for talent within a particular racing or showing area, check the sire's show record and the performance of his sons and daughters within that area.

The stud fee is an important item for many owners. Select the best stallion you can afford and try to obtain a live foal guarantee or return privilege. Make sure the stallion has a good producing record and try to see some of his offspring.

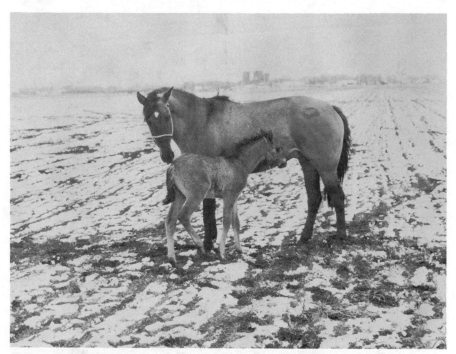

Figure 135. Although the majority of foals are spring arrivals, many youngsters come in inclement months. More care than usual is needed with these foals to guard against respiratory diseases.

175

Foaling

Prior to the time the foal is born, it receives nourishment and oxygen through the placenta via the umbilical cord. Much of its future growth potential and health are measured by the quality of diet, health care, and exercise given the mare.

Additional care is also needed at the time of foaling. The mare should have a draft-free shelter or stall, freshly bedded, or a pasture to herself. Foaling is a stressful time for the mare—and for you—even though most mares make it through with no help at all. For that percentage that

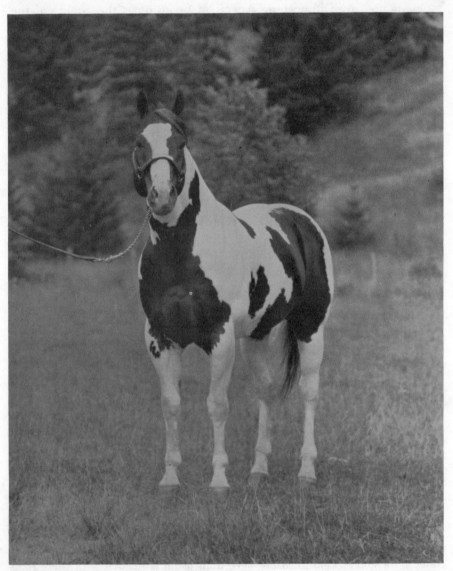

Figure 136. Paint stallion with tobiano pattern.

do need help, or for foals in need of aid, a knowledge of the foaling procedure is important.

From two to six weeks prior to birth, the mare's udder begins to enlarge. Before birth, approximately seven to ten days, the ligaments around the tail head relax and appear sunken. With this symptom, you'll also notice a dropping of the foal within the mare's belly. It gives the abdomen a fuller, lower appearance. Then, four to six days before foaling, the teats fill and milk may begin to drip from them. The final clue of impending birth is a waxy secretion on the teats. When you notice it, alert your veterinarian so he can be ready to come if you need him.

Hours before birth, the mare may go off her feed, appear listless or shift her weight back and forth. Some mares lie down, others pace nervously, break into a sweat, and paw the ground.

While you wait for the birth of the foal, stay out of the way and keep visitors to a minimum. Most mares prefer to foal at night and are irritated by commotion of any sort. Assemble the following items while you

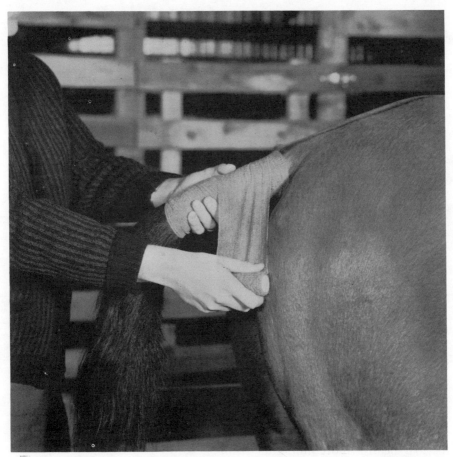

Figure 137. Wrap the tail head loosely to avoid cutting off circulation.

177

wait: hot water, mild soap, iodine for dressing the naval, clean cloths, blankets, and a tail wrap. The wrap should go on before birth to keep the hairs out of the way and free of birth fluids (Fig. 137).

The first stage of foaling begins with uterine contractions called *labor pains*. These contractions force the foal against the cervix, or opening of the uterus, and cause the bag of waters surrounding the foal to break. Many mares lie down at this time and stretch the back legs. Until the foal appears, contractions continue. *Under no circumstances try to assist the mare in foaling by pulling out the foal.* This should be done by a veterinarian ONLY if the mare is in trouble.

The presentation of the foal should come with the front feet first, heels down, and then the nose (Fig. 138). When the foal is born with the feet up, they're usually the back ones and the mare will need help in foaling. If one of the forelegs, or the umbilical cord, is twisted around the foal's neck, or if the foal is not born shortly after the mare has gone into heavy labor, CALL YOUR VETERINARIAN WITHOUT DELAY.

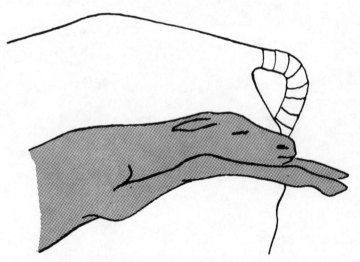

Figure 138. Correct presentation of the foal.

Foal Care

Once the foal is born, do not break or cut the cord. Through this lifeline will still flow blood needed by the foal. The mare usually ruptures the cord when she rises after birth. When the cord breaks, paint the stump with iodine.

Immediately remove any membranes covering the face, and if the weather's cold or damp, rub the foal dry with towels. Most mares will lick the foal clean a short time after rising.

Once the foal has been cared for, turn your attention to the passage of the placenta. The afterbirth should be expelled by the mare within two hours. If not expelled after six to eight hours, your veterinarian must remove it before conditions such as laminitis, pneumonia, septicemia, or metritis develop (Fig. 139). Save the placenta in a clean plastic bag so it can be examined for missing parts. Then it can be buried in lime (Fig. 140).

Back to the foal again. If healthy, he'll attempt to suckle within an hour. His arduous attempts to rise may cause you to help him to his feet, but resist the impulse. A foal gains strength through this early expenditure of energy and needs a guiding hand only toward the mare's udder. Once he's there, check to see that he's sucking correctly and that the milk is not flowing out of his mouth, thus indicating an inability to swallow.

The first few swallows of mare's milk are known as *colostrum*, rich in antibodies that guard against infections. Colostrum also has a laxative effect on the foal and is important in helping clear the intestine of *meconium*, a firm, dark fecal buildup.

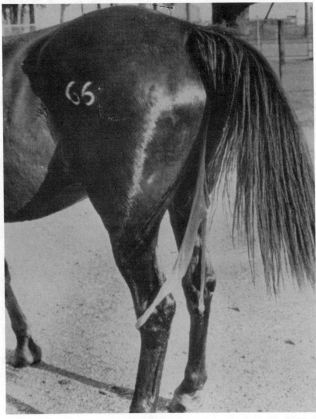

Figure 139. Retained placenta, which will have to be removed by a veterinarian.

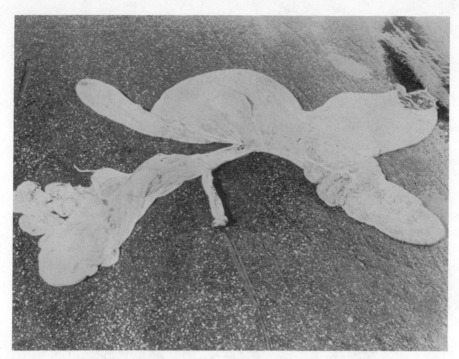

Figure 140. Complete placenta.

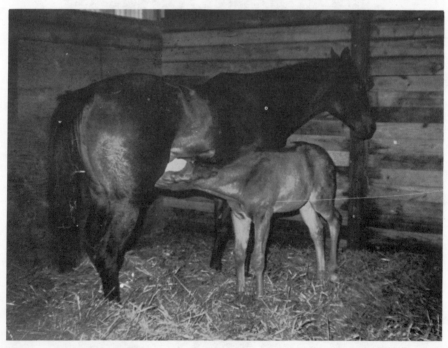

Figure 141. A foal's first meal contains the antibodies necessary to impart some immunity to disease.

Constipation

Constipation is a common problem with newborns. If the foal has nursed and not moved his bowels within five hours, your veterinarian will give him an enema. Any retained meconium can cause abdominal pains if not quickly corrected.

Diarrhea

Most foals suffer a bout of *diarrhea* when the mare comes into foal heat, the first heat after birth. This usually disappears in a few days. It's wise to call your veterinarian, just in case the cause of the problem is bacteria, and requires drugs to stop it.

Atresia Coli/Ani

The word *atresia* refers to a congenital absence of a normal passageway. With the deformity of atresia coli, the problem occurs in the colon, just before it reaches the rectum. There is an incomplete connection between two lengths of intestine.

Foals afflicted with this condition appear to be healthy after birth for a day or two. Colic then develops, along with abdominal swelling and lack of feces passage. If the amount of intestine missing is small, surgical resection may correct the problem.

Atresia ani is a similar condition requiring surgery. In many instances, the anus is totally covered with skin and this blocks normal passage of wastes.

These problems are relatively rare, and are seen by veterinarians in the Paint breed more often than in other breeds.

Hernia

A *hernia* is a rupture or incomplete closure in the wall of a cavity or abdominal wall. When such an abnormal opening is present, it allows the contents normally held back to protrude through the opening.

With an umbilical hernia, the problem is caused by an abnormally large opening in the abdominal wall. Many foals recover spontaneously from this condition by the time they are one year of age. Others need surgical correction. If a loop of intestine becomes strangulated in the hernia ring, the foal will exhibit colic symptoms. Immediate surgical correction is needed to save his life.

A scrotal hernia is noticeable at birth if the scrotum is palpated. With this type of hernia, a loop of intestine protrudes through an enlarged inguinal ring into the scrotal sac. In the majority of cases, scrotal hernia is reduced naturally without surgical correction. If strangulation occurs, immediate attention is required.

181

Pervious Urachus

The *urachus* is the tube within the umbilical cord that carried urine away before the foal was born. The word *pervious* means capable of giving passage to anything. In this case it's urine. The newborn drips urine from the unwithered urachus at the navel stump.

Usually within a few days, the condition clears up spontaneously. If not, surgical correction is required. Don't wait for the urachus to wither when you notice urine dripping: call your veterinarian. If germs should enter the urachus, they'll travel into the bladder and cause inflammation.

Septicemia

Septicemia means the presence in the blood of pus-forming organisms. These bacteria infect the foal while in the uterus or during the first few days of life. After birth, entry into the bloodstream is made through a contaminated navel or via body wounds.

The signs of septicemia are a rise in temperature, disinterest in nursing, inability to stand, and either a sudden or slow decline until death. The symptoms differ with the type of bacteria causing the infection.

Swelling of the joints, along with a temperature rise, is called *navel* or *joint ill*. The bacteria in the blood localize in one or more joints and produce pus, thereby causing extreme tenderness. Lameness and soreness may be constant, or disappear and reappear. If the disease is acute, the foal will discontinue nursing and move with apparent pain. The navel cord may have pus draining from it or have a crusty, enlarged appearance. Diarrhea may be present in some cases.

Diseased foals need antibiotic treatment immediately. It's most successful if started in the early stages of the disease. Because the foals become dehydrated, they also need supportive therapy (vitamins, electrolyte solutions, and often, blood transfusions).

Some afflicted foals appear to recover and develop into normal, healthy-looking yearlings. But if the illness has been prolonged, and the joints enlarged at the time treatment began, the foal may have joint cartilage erosion. Such youngsters are not often successful in a racing career.

Prevention of septicemia relies heavily on good management procedures and immediate care of wounds and the navel stump. Disinfect and clean the foaling pen with steam or a strong chemical disinfectant. Replace bedding after foaling and disinfect all water and feed buckets.

After birth, the mare's udder and hindquarters should be cleaned. Proper care of the umbilical stump with the application of iodine or antiseptic will guard against entrance of bacterial bloodstream invasion. If the foal is born in cold or wet weather, keep mare and foal inside. Exposure while young may predispose the foal to respiratory and systemic infections that could prove fatal. Consult with your veterinarian and begin the foal on a periodic, regular immunization program. Also be sure to keep the mare on her vaccination program, both before and after foaling.

Immunization Program

To protect the foal, the mare should have a tetanus toxoid booster within one month prior to foaling, assuming she has been on a tetanus toxoid program. If this is done, the foal will not need an injection of tetanus antitoxin shortly after birth, because he will receive it in the mare's colostrum.

The vaccination program for the foal is as follows:

2½ to 3 months of age	1st tetanus toxoid
	1st influenza vaccination
	1st rhinopneumonitis
3½ to 4 months of age	2nd tetanus toxoid
	2nd influenza
	2nd rhinopneumonitis
yearling	booster of each above

The Eastern and Western encephalomyelitis vaccine can also be given at the above ages, but if the mare has been on a constant vaccination program, many veterinarians prefer to wait until the spring of yearling age to vaccinate.

Premature and Orphan Foals

The *premature foal* is handicapped in proportion to the number of weeks he is premature. If born too early, his system will not have developed to the point of adjusting, and he will not survive.

Breathing is one of the biggest problems facing the premature foal. His chest muscles and cough reflex are weak, thus decreasing the inflation power of his lungs. His inability to cough and expel phlegm also makes the foal susceptible to respiratory problems such as pneumonia. Many premies have a difficult time starting or continuing breathing because the respiratory response center of their brain is underdeveloped and unable to correctly balance oxygen and carbon dioxide in the blood and lungs. Maintaining respiration is also a result of less blood volume than present in a full-term foal.

In his weakened condition, the premature foal is usually unable to suckle properly and take in the required amount of nutrition. He's often unable to receive colostrum, a fact that seriously affects his vulnerability to disease. His own tissues and organs are so underdeveloped that he cannot produce the enzymes and antibodies he needs to protect himself.

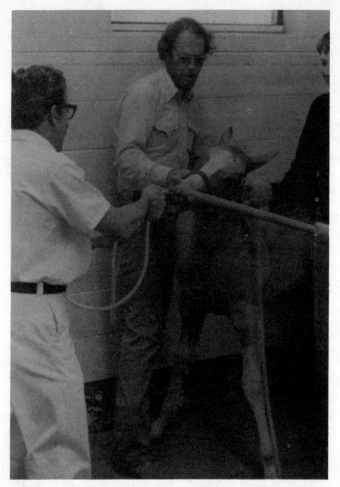

Figure 142. Begin worming a foal at an early age to ensure maximum growth and good health.

In short, the premature foal has to fight for his life.

The *orphaned foal*, on the other hand, has a greater chance for survival with the proper nursing care and attention. If the mare is alive, but shows hostility to the foal, there are some methods you can use for permitting the foal to nurse. Try tying the mare while the foal nurses: some mares will, in time lose their hostility after they become accustomed to the procedure. If you have to keep them permanently separated, and the mare tries to kick or bite the foal when you bring him to nurse, then twitch her or hold up a leg until the foal is finished.

Should the mare be dead or unable to produce milk, our major concern is whether the foal received colostrum if he was able to nurse a time or two. Some breeding farms can supply you with frozen colos-

184

trum. If you have trouble obtaining it, your veterinarian will usually put the foal on an intensive program of antibiotics, and may give blood to impart some immunity to disease.

Feeding the foal is time-consuming and difficult for many owners. Finding a nurse mare is the best solution, but often out of the question. The next alternative is to find a commercial mare milk that agrees with the foal and is tolerated by his system. Once again, your veterinarian will be able to suggest several brands, and a feeding schedule.

After about twenty-one days of being on a formula, you can provide the foal with leafy alfalfa hay in unlimited quantities. Grain should be offered at the same time in the form of steamed, rolled oats mixed with a vitamin and mineral supplement, and bone meal at half a pound per one hundred pounds. The meal should be increased as the foal matures.

Providing green pasture and companions to run with is also an essential part of being a foster parent. Horses raised alone develop an antisocial attitude toward other horses when they become adults. Later, pastured as an adult with others of their kind, they turn either timid or aggressive in nature. This is because they've missed an important part of social development in growing up alone.

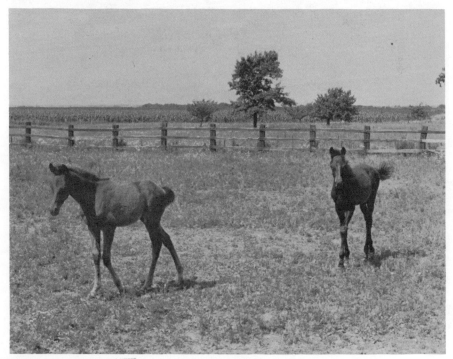

Figure 143. Orphaned foals do better with company than alone.

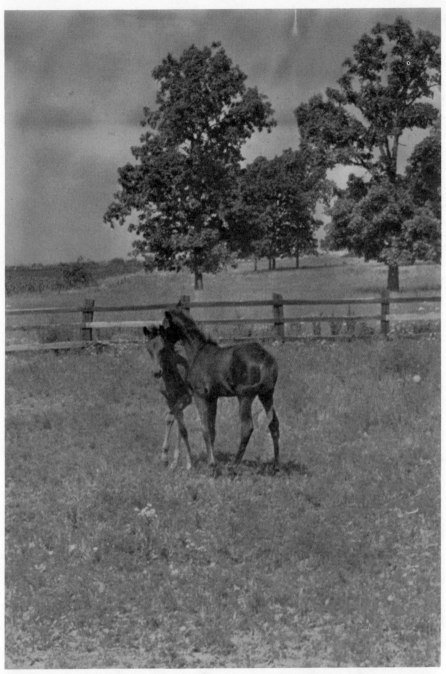

Figure 144. To develop a social, well-rounded personality, a foal needs play-mates of his own age to grow with.

Weaning and Drying Up

Weaning is a sad and traumatic time in a mare and foal's life. When to separate depends on several factors. The first is whether the dam has been rebred. If she has, the foal may be weaned from four to six months of age. Early weaning saves the mare's strength, since nursing one foal and carrying another are quite a burden. Early weaning may also take place if the mare must be returned to work, or if either mare or foal is sick. Should you decide to let nature take care of the problem, the mare will usually have the foal weaned at about a year.

The quickest way to wean a foal is separation from the sight and sound of mother. Unfortunately, many horses will become so distressed at this sudden loss, they're apt to injury themselves trying to escape confinement. Should you choose this cold-turkey method, be sure there are no sharp objects in the stall or pen that could injure either horse. Tranquilizers may be a help in quieting the mare.

A second, though longer and calmer method is to place the mare and foal in adjoining stalls. Often another foal is placed in the stall or confinement paddock to make the separation easier on both foals. Extra attention should be given at separation time and exercise time for both mare and foal maintained or increased.

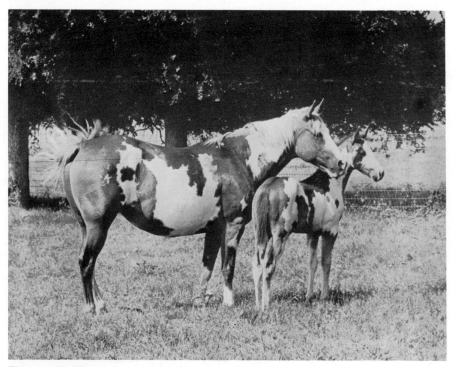

Figure 145. Typical American Paint mare and her foal with an overo pattern.

187

When the mare is taken from the foal, she is still producing large quantities of milk. Production is stimulated by the foal's sucking and head bumping on the udder. So after the foal is taken away, be sure to *avoid* massaging the udder (in the mistaken hope of milking the mare dry) or the supply will continue. Milk production will halt in time when pressure inside the bag reaches a point to terminate new production.

In most mares, udder pressure causes heat and swelling. If she appears to be in pain, and the swelling extends to the abdominal wall, call your veterinarian. He can prescribe drugs to reduce the problem. Keep exercising the mare during this period and reduce the grain for about a week. This may help slow up milk production.

Castration

What age is best for castration? The answer varies from foalhood—particularly if the colt shows no conformational gift for showing, breeding, or racing—to whenever the colt gets too rank to handle. If your colt has a nice disposition, then you may want to wait until he's a year or two old. The longer you wait, the more development of stallion characteristics he'll have. This means—in most cases—a thicker neck and muscular body, and a more aggressive nature.

10

Emergency First Aid

When you're suddenly confronted with an emergency situation, it's frightening. You're faced with having to quickly analyze how serious is the problem, how fast a veterinarian can get to your horse, and if there's anything you can do to aid the animal while you're waiting. Handling such a problem calls for calmness and a basic knowledge of first aid. If you have these two things, chances are you can prevent some complications from developing during that critical waiting period. You can also make the veterinarian's job easier when he does get there if you've acted promptly and correctly.

RESPIRATION, PULSE, AND TEMPERATURE

Supply your veterinarian with the results of respiration, pulse, and temperature at the time of the initial call for help, and when he arrives on the scene. It's vital for him to know if there's been a rise or fall in any of these body signs.

Respiration
Respiration is how often the horse takes air into the lungs (inspiration) and expels it (expiration) per minute. The normal respiratory rate is eight to sixteen times per minute if the horse is resting. After severe exercise the rate might be thirty to forty times or more per minute.

189

To take the respiration rate, get a stopwatch and count the number of in-and-out motions made by the rib cage. You can also put your hand on the ribs or flank and feel the breathing movements.

Pulse

When the heart pumps blood through the arteries, there is an intermittent wave, or *pulse*, that can be felt. A resting horse has a pulse rate of thirty-six to forty times per minute. It increases with exercise, injury, stress, or excitement. After exercise, the rate could reach one hundred, which is normal. If the horse is calm, however, that rate would be cause for alarm.

To take the pulse, locate the large artery that runs around the inner side of the jaw (Fig. 146). Grasp the jaw between your thumb and forefingers so the pulse can be felt under your fingers. Check it with the second hand of your watch. If the horse objects to this method, use the artery on the inside of the elbow of the foreleg.

Temperature

The normal temperature range for the calm, resting horse is 99.5°–100.5°, with variations caused by sex, age, day, season, climate, mating, and outside temperature. In young foals, two months of age and under, the *normal* temperature is 101.5°.

To take the temperature, buy a rectal thermometer from your veterinarian or livestock supply store. Get a maximum registering rectal thermometer of heavy construction. As with a human thermometer, shake down the mercury, lubricate the bulb with Vaseline, and place it gently in the rectum. Have the horse held while you're inserting it and firmly hold in place three minutes for accurate reading.

PROBLEM WARNING SIGNS

Quite often an emergency situation is preceded by symptoms. If you miss the warning signs of possible, imminent trouble, you could find yourself with a real emergency.

1. Change in appetite.
2. Fast or slow, continuous bleeding from any opening.
3. Change in bowel habits, such as diarrhea, constipation, or in bowel movement color.
4. Sudden change in behavior.
5. Breathing difficulties such as heavy, fast or shallow respiration.
6. Change in the texture or shine of the coat.
7. Nasal discharge.

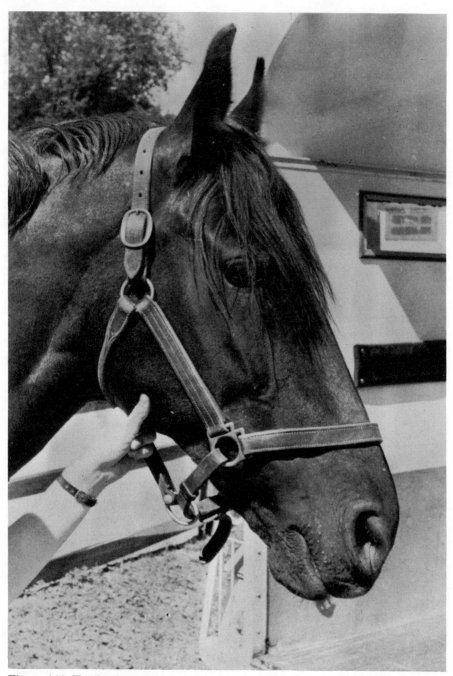

Figure 146. To check the pulse, grasp the horse in the manner shown and time the pulse with a stopwatch.

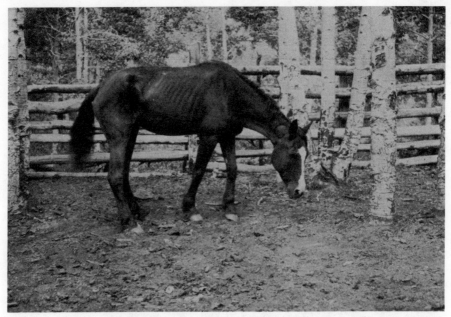

Figure 147. Staggering and weight loss are indications of a problem. In this case the horse has symptoms of plant poisoning.

8. Difficulty with urination or defecation.
9. Convulsions or shaking.
10. Abnormal swelling anywhere on the body.
11. Elevated temperature.
12. Inability to rise from a recumbent position in the stall or pasture.
13. Abnormal sweating or lack of it in hot weather.
14. Excessive fatigue for three days or more.
15. Loss of sensation in an area.
16. Pain in any part of the body.
17. Paralysis of a part.
18. Stiffness in a limb.
19. Sudden weight loss.
20. Loss of vision, partial or complete.

FIRST-AID KIT SUPPLIES

First-aid supplies should be kept in the stable and in the car when you trailer. It also is wise to carry a portable packet when you're riding the trail.

You will note that the following list is simple, minus a lot of wound powders, caustic liquid wound preparations, and commercial ointments. The list contains just enough to handle most emergencies until the veterinarian arrives. Above all, it ensures that any wound will not be contaminated or injured by the application of caustic (burning), irritating substances that retard healing. Basic supplies include:

epsom salts
vinegar
baking powder
sterile gauze pads
Vaseline
furacin or antibiotic ointment
adhesive tape
scissors, tweezers
gallon of distilled water
rectal thermometer
elastic bandages
wire clippers
pliers for removing nails in the foot
rubber flushing syringe for squirting saline solution
rolls of cotton for immobilizing and wrapping leg wounds
fly repellant

EMERGENCY SITUATIONS

Burns
1. Call your veterinarian.
2. Acid burn:bathe with one teaspoon baking soda dissolved in a pint of warm water.
3. Alkali burn: bathe with equal solution of vinegar and warm water.
4. Cover with sterile dressing.
5. Keep the horse blanketed and offer water.

Choking
1. Call your veterinarian.
2. Massage the esophagus on the underside of the throat in stroking motions toward the chest.
3. Give a mild tranquilizer if you're experienced.
4. Withhold all food and water until the object is dislodged.

Heat Exhaustion
1. Call your veterinarian.
2. Cool the body with cold hose spray or pack body with ice. If

delirium occurs, put ice on the head. Pack the feet to prevent laminitis.
3. Keep out of the sun and do not work.

Heat exhaustion is a common problem during summer months or when the horse is tied in the sun or confined to a poorly ventilated stable after heavy work. The cause is overheating, rather than the direct effect of the sun's rays.

The first signs of sunstroke or heat exhaustion are stumbling, a refusal to work, weakness, and refusal to eat. Sweating often stops and the skin is dry. If the horse is forced to work after initial signs develop, convulsions and collapse will follow. The temperature may rise to 106°–110° or higher. The pulse rate is accelerated and the heart may be felt pounding.

Horses that are cooled and live for a few hours will usually recover: those that collapse and are delirious usually die within two hours. Animals with a high temperature accompanied by weakness and delirium are also not likely to live.

Snakebite
1. Call your veterinarian.
2. Keep the horse quiet and apply ice packs and cold water over the area to prevent swelling.
3. If you're on the trail when this happens, walk the horse home slowly.
4. Most horses recover without treatment, but the period is much longer without supportive therapy.

Shock
1. Call your veterinarian.
2. Keep the horse warm.
3. Attend to any external bleeding or wounds.
4. If lying down, move the tongue to the bars to ensure the horse is breathing well.
5. If the horse is standing, keep water available.

Wounds
Wounds may be classified as *open*, with the skin surface and/or underlying tissues and structures torn and injured, or *closed*, as with a bruise. Open wounds are a portal of entry for bacteria and subsequent infection of the wound. The aim of treatment with an open wound is to have it closed quickly, without infection, and with as little excess proud flesh as possible.

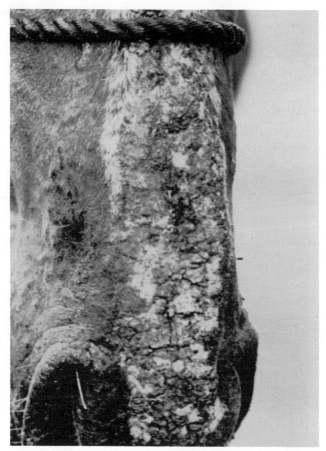

Figure 148. The sun can also burn the white or pink, unpigmented areas of a horse's face. Provide shade for these animals when they are out in pasture.

Open wounds may be subclassified into (1) abrasions, (2) lacerations, (3) avulsed wounds, and (4) puncture wounds (Fig. 149). Each is treated according to its appearance, depth, and involvement with deeper structures, plus its potential site for infection and healing.

Abrasions

Abrasions are breaks in the surface layer of the skin by rubbing, scraping, or falling. The area has spotty bleeding, is highly contaminated, and may be slow to heal.

1. Wash the injury with warm water and mild soap.
2. Remove foreign matter and dirt.
3. Do not apply any substance to the wound if the abrasion is extensive. Call your veterinarian.
4. If the abrasion is mild, apply Vaseline to keep tissues from drying.

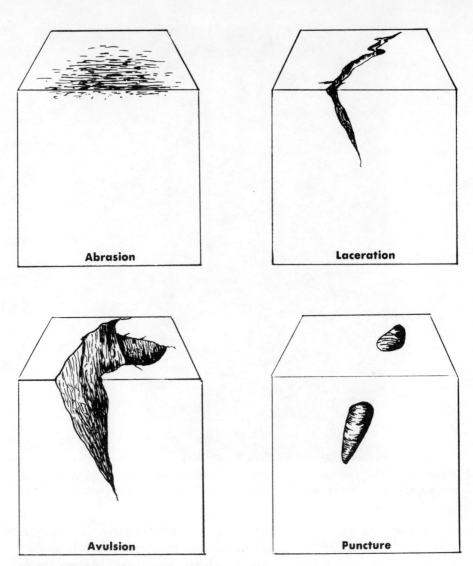

Figure 149. Wound examples of skin sections.

Laceration

A *laceration* usually has cleanly cut edges that do not gape open. There is generally little tissue damage, and pain and bleeding vary according to the depth and extent of the wound. In serious cases, there is damage to underlying tissues and organs.

1. Stop bleeding by applying direct pressure over the site. Use gauze pads over the area and wrap tightly (Fig. 150 and 151).
2. If you cannot wrap the site, or do not have gauze available, use hand pressure until your veterinarian arrives.

196

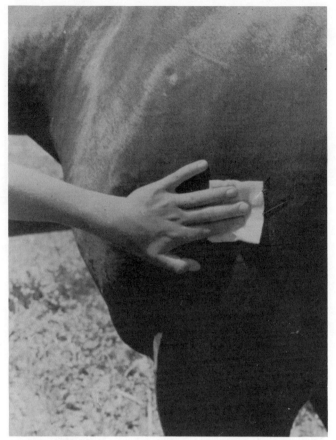

Figure 150. Apply direct pressure over a bleeding wound with a gauze pad to staunch the flow of blood and keep bacteria out of the wound.

3. If the wound is severe, keep the horse blanketed during cold months.
4. Bright red blood indicates that an artery has been cut. It will need to be surgically tied off.
5. Most nonarterial cuts stop bleeding of their own accord in fifteen to thirty minutes, so don't be alarmed at the amount of dark blood issuing from the wound.
6. Any wound one and one-half inches or more in depth needs veterinary attention.
7. Flush the wound with warm saline solution. This is made of two teaspoons salt in one quart boiled water.
8. Cover the wound with a sterile dressing.
9. Any wound over twenty-four hours old will be infected and the tissues so swollen they usually can't be stitched.

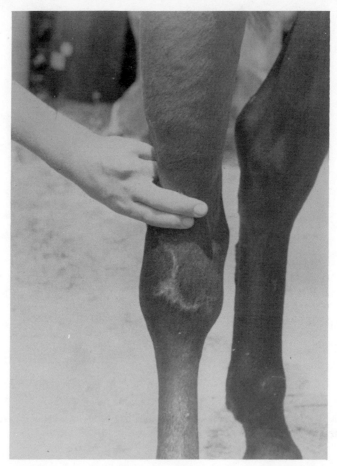

Figure 151. Use finger pressure above a wound to cut down the flow of blood from a wound until veterinary aid arrives.

Avulsed Wounds

Avulsed wounds are those with pieces of skin and tissue missing. They are difficult, if not impossible to suture, especially below the knee, and are usually left open to heal (Fig. 152).

1. Call your veterinarian.
2. Treat as for a laceration with warm saline solution and cover with a sterile dressing.
3. Do not run water over a laceration or avulsed wound, since this encourages swelling and later development of proud flesh. Limit wet applications and do not handle the wound any more than necessary.

198

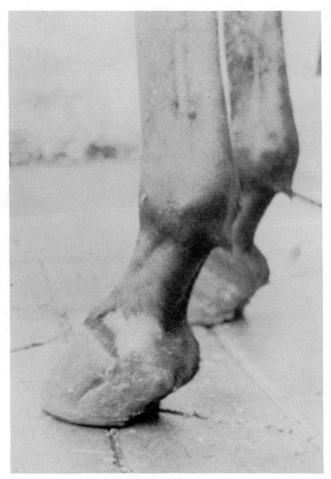

Figure 152. Healed avulsed wound showing damage to the coronary band and subsequent deformation of the hoof below the wound. Note the failure of hair to recover the wound site.

Puncture Wounds

Puncture wounds penetrate the tissues, body cavities, or feet and carry infectious organisms with them. They're extremely dangerous and prompt veterinary attention is necessary. Do not hesitate to call for help regardless of the size of the penetrating object, since a tetanus antitoxin shot must be given.

1. If the object penetrates the abdomen, keep the horse still and cross-tie him if you must leave to call for help.
2. If the object penetrates the chest cavity, don't remove the object: let the veterinarian do it. If you attempt removal, air can enter the chest and collapse the lungs. Plug the area around the object

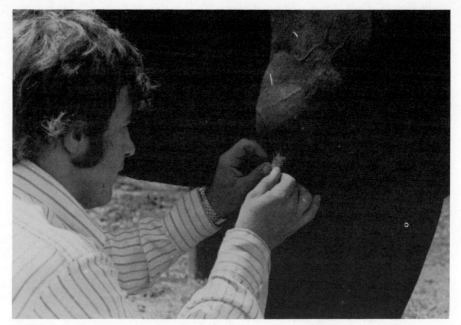

Figure 153. Puncture wounds need immediate attention because of the large number of bacteria and dirt carried into the wound.

with large pieces of gauze to seal off air entry routes.

3. If the foot is penetrated, the entry hole usually seals over and must be professionally opened to permit drainage. Wrap the foot to prevent further contamination and wait for aid.
4. Flush all puncture wounds with a saline solution.
5. Keep the horse still and warm.

Bruises

Bruises, or *contusions,* damage the underlying tissue and bony area. Often, as with kicks to a nonfleshy area, there may be a fracture to treat as well as damage tissue. Sometimes a blood vessel will rupture and cause a cold, soft swelling called a *hematoma.* This should not be lanced, or drained, but treated by your veterinarian.

1. Treat a bruise with ice packs or cold water and repeat often for the first twenty-four hours.
2. Forty-eight hours after the injury, apply heat to bring blood to the area.
3. Use hot epsom salt packs and gentle massage, along with linaments, if advised by your veterinarian.

How Do Wounds Heal?

Wounds should heal the way nature intended, without interference

200

from manmade irritants or harsh antiseptics. These solutions damage the tissues and retard healing, rather than help it.

Immediately after the skin and tissue are injured, nature seeks to heal the injury with *first-intention healing*. This objective is best accomplished with veterinary suturing (Fig. 154). First-intention healing is basically restoration of the tissues.

With an uncomplicated, relatively uncontaminated wound, the edges become "glued" together by substances in the blood clotting at the incision line. The "glue" holds the wound together on the surface, while the stronger connective tissue cells multiply.

Then the fibroblasts and small capillary buds grow into the blood clot, or coagulum, and replace them. During this time, the skin cells are growing to bridge the incision line.

If the skin edges are not closed sutures, and the edges of the wound are rubbed or irritated by harsh antiseptics, the wound must close by *second-intention healing* or *granulation*. Granulation tissue is composed of capillary vessels and fibroblasts. The difference between first and second intention healing is that in second intention, *growth starts from the inner or bottom depths* of the wound, rather than from the edges.

When the tissue fills in the wound, it produces a rough, insensitive red tissue that bleeds easily. After the granulation tissue has filled in the

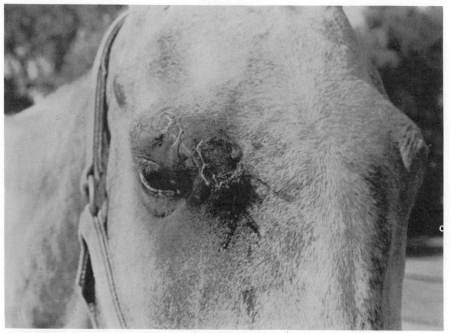

Figure 154. Wounds need immediate attention if they are to heal properly and not develop secondary complications.

201

wound gap, the surface is thick enough to prevent bacterial invasion.

Gradually the epithelial cells of the skin begin to multiply and bridge the gap filled in by granulation tissue. If too much tissue develops during the course of healing, it is called *proud flesh* (Fig. 155). This must be surgically removed to allow closure or proper healing by epithelial tissue. If you can keep pressure over the wound and limit its movement, this will deter some granulation tissue development.

Healing Failures

Some wounds fail to heal, or take a long time to heal because there is excessive motion of the area. In some areas, the wound breaks open and the attempt of the body at healing must start again. Wounds also fail to heal because foreign bodies are left in the wound and cause a discharge.

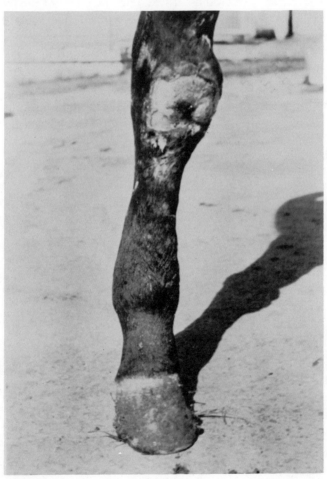

Figure 155. Severe deformation of the hock due to an untreated wound that formed proud flesh.

Harsh disinfectants or soap can retard healing, as can poor drainage of accumulated tissue exudates. Other setbacks include infection, insect interference, summer sores, parasitic infestation, and regeneration fatigue. *Regeneration fatigue* usually occurs in wounds where there is a loss of a lot of tissue. Surgical stimulation is needed to allow the wound to begin healing again.

Fractures
1. Call your veterinarian immediately.
2. Treat the wound, if there is one.
3. Take two pillows and bind the leg tightly. Then apply a broomstick, two boards, or any rigid object and wrap tightly.
4. Keep the horse still and warm.

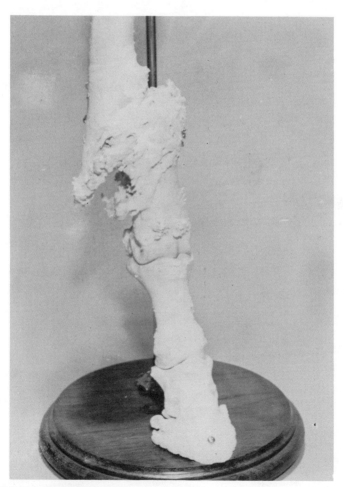

Figure 156. Nature healed this cannon bone fracture and built calcium deposits to hold the two ends together.

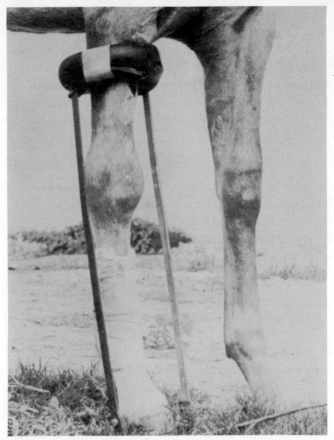

Figure 157. Some cannon bone fractures can be set and the horse returned to serviceability.

Types of Fractures

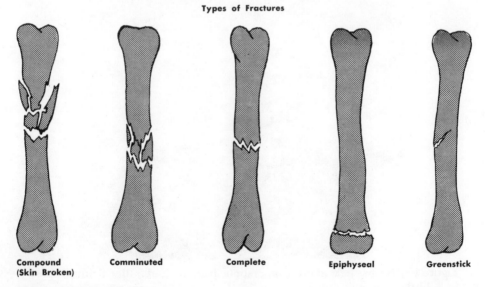

Compound (Skin Broken) Comminuted Complete Epiphyseal Greenstick

Figure 158. Types of fractures.

Bandaging

When you bandage a leg wound, cover the wound first with a sterile dressing and then place a layer of cotton around the leg. Take an elastic bandage and firmly (not tightly) wind it above, over, and below the wound to control bleeding.

When you bandage for swelling, strain, or sprain, wrap first with cotton and start the elastic bandage just under the knee. Secure the end in a turn of the bandage and continue to wrap tightly *down* the leg. The ankle and part of the pastern should be covered before you start up again. Secure the wrap with a velcro strap or a wrap tie. If you use safety pins to keep the bandage closed, fold over part of the bandage and put adhesive tape around it.

When you wrap, keep the bandage flat and don't let any twists or wrinkles occur. Change the bandage daily, since it relaxes when swelling goes down and offers little support to the leg when loose.

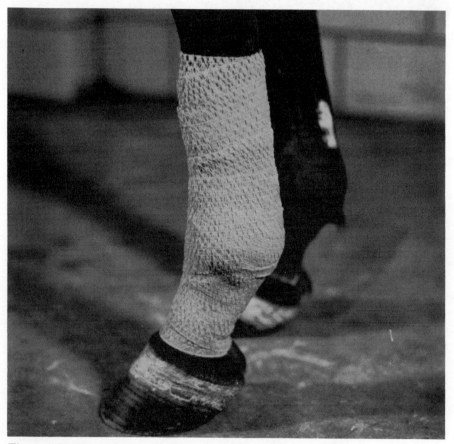

Figure 159. Example of a bandage used to support the fetlock area.

205

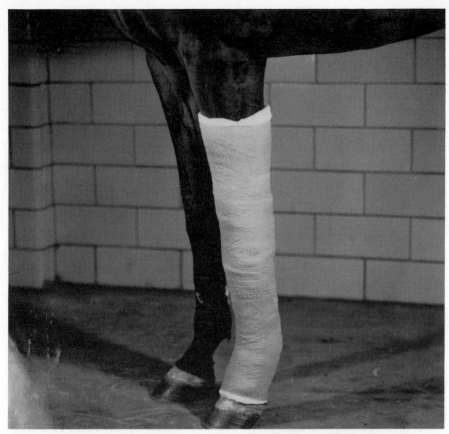

Figure 160. This bandage is used to hold a dressing in place rather than give support to one specific area of the leg.

Strain and Sprain

A *strain* is overstretching or overexerting some part of the musculature to a harmful degree.

A *sprain* is a joint injury in which some of the fibers of a supporting ligament are ruptured, resulting in bleeding, heat, swelling, and pain. The severity of the sprain is directly proportional to the numbers of fibers torn. This injury heals with scar tissue and may cause a predisposition to weakness and recurring injury if the horse is worked too hard in the future.

Veterinary attention should be immediate. Reduce the swelling until help comes by soaking the part in cold water or by applying cold packs. Apply DMSO for five to seven days (under veterinary advisement) and keep bandaged. If swelling returns after you've taken off the bandages, rebandage at night only—not when exercising the horse—and keep on for another four to seven days.

206

11

Trailering Safety

Pulling your horse with minimum stress on your tow vehicle and maximum safety for your rig depends on three interdependent factors. The first is selecting the proper tow vehicle and trailer; the second knowing how to load with the least trauma; and the third, understanding how to haul without creating problems for your horses or other drivers.

SELECTING YOUR RIG

Let's start the selection of the rig with the *tow vehicle*, since it supplies the power to pull the trailer and get it out of trouble on the highway. What, exactly, is a good tow vehicle? It's a *safe* car, four-wheel drive, or pickup designed to meet the strain of pulling thousands of pounds without breaking down, or creating oscillation (fishtailing) of the trailer. Sounds pretty basic, doesn't it? Well, unfortunately, there are far too many tow vehicles on the highway that don't meet basic safety requirements, mostly because the driver isn't aware of minimum safety standards. They are:

1. The car must be no smaller than a lightweight classification, and preferably heavier.

2. It should have a *minimum* engine size of 360 CID 2-barrel V8.

3. The *gross vehicle weight* (the total weight of the tow vehicle with passengers or cargo) should be twice the weight of the trailer it has to pull.

4. If used in mountains, the tow vehicle must be three times the weight of the trailer.

5. It should be capable of pulling the specified loaded weight of the trailer (the gross towing weight). This information can be obtained from the vehicle manufacturer or in the dealer's specifications book.

6. The greater the distance in inches from the rear axle to the rear bumper, the less stable the rig. The theory behind this is that every car is supposed to travel as a balanced load with the front and rear bumper the same height from the ground. When you put on a hitch and trailer, and possibly install air shocks to "equalize" all this weight, what happens?

Just like an unbalanced teeter totter, the front end comes up and the rear goes down. So the farther over the rear axle the car hangs, the more the back of the vehicle sinks, and the more fishtailing you get with the trailer. There's also a significant increase in wear and stress on the rear tires and axle, hence the possibility of a breakdown while towing.

7. The car must have a *gross axle weight rating* high enough to support the weight of the hitch and tongue weight. You cannot exceed the total allowable load on the rear axle without damaging the system. The GAWR is listed on the dealer's specifications sheet.

8. The car must not be smaller in length than the trailer.

9. It should be equipped with *leaf springs* rather than coils, since the latter tend to break more easily under heavy loads and road vibration. There should be a minimum combined number of four leaf springs in the front and six to eight in the rear to support the load.

10. Fluid drive transmissions are made for a noiseless ride, not towing loads. Automobiles with such transmissions are not suitable for towing a heavy load over long distances, several times a week.

11. The car should be equipped with a *heavy-duty towing package*. This includes a Class III Equalizing hitch, extra-duty cooling package, heavy flasher, five wire wiring harness, increased axle ration of 3.45:1, heavy front and rear springs and shocks, extra-duty cooling system, heavy alternator and battery, and automatic transmission.

12. A four-wheel drive with a long wheel base is excellent for towing, since it has a sturdier suspension system and frame. It is also designed to pull out of mud and snow, and has a short rear overhang for more stability.

13. A three quarter-ton and a one-ton pickup truck are high safety margin towers that are designed for hard work, rather than passenger comfort. They can be equipped to haul over eight thousand pounds and can pull from the rear or from the truck bed (a gooseneck hitchup).

Safety Hints

1. Add a deflector to the tailpipe to keep fumes from passing into the trailer.

2. Install wide mudflaps on rear tires to cut down on mud and gravel spray on the trailer.

3. Use the best tires on the market for wearability and increased safety.

4. Don't haul with a full-car passenger load over long distances.

5. Avoid hauling with the air conditioner on, since it strains the engine.

6. Use cruise control to avoid engine strain and conserve gas.

7. Don't pump your brakes when you stop.

8. To avoid lugging the engine when driving uphill, use downshift #1. If additional power is needed, even though you're rolling up at a good pace, go to #2.

9. When going downhill, shift into #1 to avoid burning out the brakes. Be careful when doing this, since you can jerk your whole rig.

The Hitch

Trailer safety experts blame approximately eighty percent of all trailer accidents on the hitch. This is an astounding statistic when you consider that the problems range from mere selection errors to failure to latch the couple.

For towing live weight, you need the heaviest, safest hitch available, a Class III Equalizing hitch (Figs. 161 and 162) designed to handle up to five thousand pounds when pulled by a car, and up to seven thousand pounds with a pickup truck. Anything over seven thousand pounds is pulled by a gooseneck coupler.

When you order your hitch from a trailer service center or hitch installation dealer, you'll need to know the *tongue weight* and height of your trailer and the *ball size*. The ball size must correspond to the size of the receptacle on the trailer tongue or the trailer will become uncoupled while towing.

When the hitch is installed, it should be both *welded* and *bolted* to the car frame. It should also be installed at the *correct height* from the ground. It cannot be higher or lower than the horizontally balanced height of the trailer. Even though properly balanced when you leave the hitch installation dealer, your load can become unbalanced by where you place your cargo. Keep all weight in the car ahead of the rear axle and about sixty percent of it ahead of the trailer axles.

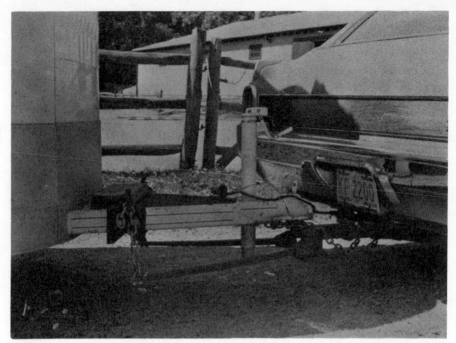

Figure 161. Correct hitch set-up with equalizer bars in place and a Class III hitch.

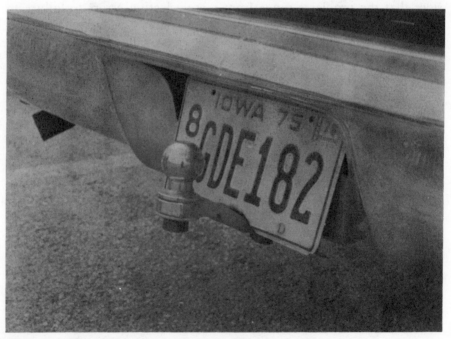

Figure 162. The hitch is too lightweight for towing live weight.

Trailer Models

Trailer models range from a single-horse to a six-horse and larger. This discussion will deal with single- to four-horse models.

The *single-horse trailer* can be ordered with or without a dressing room, and with most of the options available on a two-horse model. It is easy to tow and maneuver and costs less for the one-horse owner.

Many single trailers are manufactured with only one axle and no brakes, a definite safety problem. All trailers carrying live weight should have brakes, since a car is not designed to effectively stop itself, plus the added weight of a horse and trailer. A single axle with two tires is not as safe as a four-tired, double-axle trailer. If you have a blowout with only two tires, the trailer usually tips over.

The *two-horse model* gives you the option of carrying a second horse and a better resale value. It can be ordered as a *tandem* (horses pulled side by side), or as an *in-line* (horses pulled one behind the other) (Fig. 163). Tandems are popular because they're compact and easy to back, while the in-lines afford good visibility while being towed and better weight distribution.

Either type is available as an enclosed *van* or an open sided *stock* trailer (Figs. 164 and 165). For long hauls and cold climates, the van has comfort and luxury, taller head dimensions, and more length and width of stall.

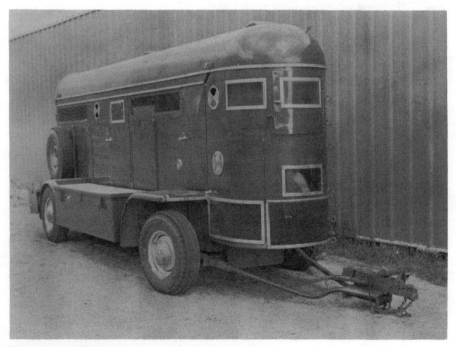

Figure 163. A deluxe two-horse in-line trailer.

211

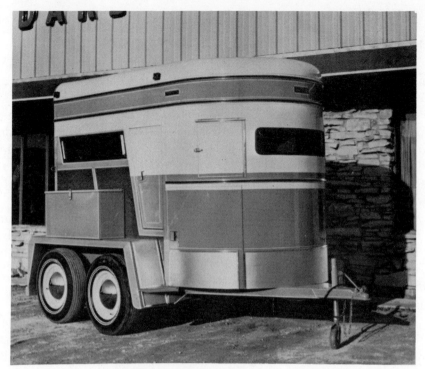

Figure 164. Two-horse trailer equipped with convenient feed box over fender and sliding side windows, both useful options.

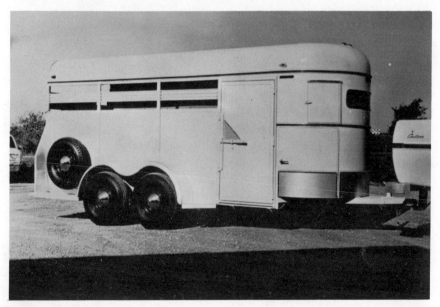

Figure 165. Deluxe four-horse stock trailer with full escape door, feed door, and tack storage.

The stock trailer is less expensive and very serviceable for short hauls and warm-weather climates.

Options

There are many options available in trailer models that can be classified as safety or convenience options. For safety, order the following:

1. A full escape door, rather than a half-door.
2. Front windows to lighten the interior, give better balance because of visibility, and to relieve boredom.
3. Side vents or windows to circulate air.
4. Side or rear curtains to keep out rain or snow.
5. Padded chest, sides, rear, and head areas.
6. Floor mats rather than straw over bare wood.
7. Interior lights.
8. Extra height and/or width for a large horse.
9. Full running lights on top and sides.
10. A spare tire, tool kit, and flares.
11. A carpeted or rubber ramp to avoid slipping and cut down noise.

To make your horses comfortable, loading easier, and extend the life

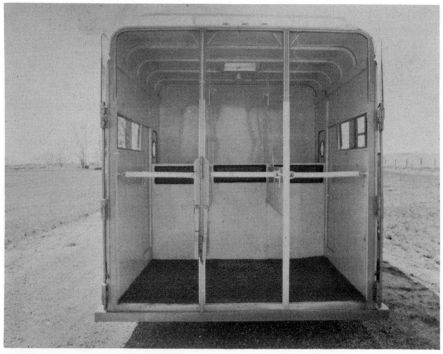

Figure 166. A well-lighted and ventilated three-horse trailer. The straight rump bars discourage "sitting" as on rump chains.

of the trailer, you can order from a large number of convenience options.

1. Gravel guards across the front and over the fenders.

2. A ramp gate assist to make lifting easier.

3. Metal or rubber kickplates in the stalls.

4. Undercoating.

5. A rubber suspension system that is offered by some manufacturers to give a vibration-free ride.

6. A movable center partition to allow easy loading.

7. An extra height ramp or doors for tall horses that hang over a standard height rear closure.

Brake Systems

Electric brakes on a trailer are activated by an electrical impulse that is sent from the car brakes (which are hydraulic) back to your trailer brakes. When the rig is wired, the car's hydraulic system is bypassed and the electrical system hooked up to work from the car brakes, but not with them.

This means it takes a few seconds longer for the braking impulse to reach and stop the trailer after the car brakes have been applied. The strength of the impulse is controlled by a knob on the control box that is mounted under the dash or on the steering wheel of the car. If your car brakes should fail, the entire rig can be stopped with the trailer brakes.

Maintenance on this system is relatively easy, but does involve frequent checks to see that the wiring is not coming loose from the molding, is not damaged, or not loose in the plugs. Attention should be paid to periodically replacing the car brake light fuse. If this goes, so do the trailer brakes.

Hydraulic surge brakes (Fig. 167) operate independently from the car. All you have to do is have the car wired for lights and you're ready to haul. There's no wiring for brakes. The hydraulic surge system operates on the principle that, when the braking car slows down, the forward pressure of the trailer on the car hitch activates and applies brake pressure on the trailer. The system utilizes hydraulic fluid, rather than electricity.

The biggest advantage of a surge hookup is that you can use more than one tow vehicle to haul the trailer. Its disadvantage is that the brakes are activated when the rig is driven downhill or backed up an incline. This is particularly treacherous when the roads are steep, icy, or slippery. Some states with mountainous terrain have outlawed the surge system as unsafe.

Hydraulic brakes are hooked up to and operated with the car's hydraulic brakes as one simultaneous system. There's no delay and no independent braking action.

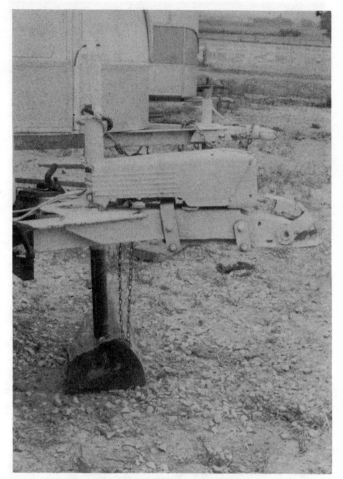

Figure 167. Hydraulic surge brake system.

The disadvantage of this system is that, in the event of a breakdown, the brake lines rupture, and the car is without braking action. Should the car brakes ever fail, the entire rig is without stopping power.

Maintenance for both hydraulic brakes and hydraulic surge brakes includes keeping a periodic watch on the level of the hydraulic fluid, and seeing that the lines are cleaned to prevent clogging. The brake lines should also be inspected for holes and inclosed in molded channels.

Trailer Maintenance

Regular cleaning and inspection of all working parts raises your safety margin on the road. Use the manufacturer's instructions, or maintain your trailer according to the following points of care.

1. Lubrication of all hinges with silicone spray is necessary to keep

215

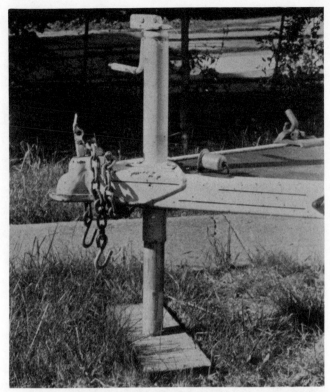

Figures 168 and 169. Take off the wheel when you tow and park your trailer. The trailer in Figure 169 was hauled with the wheel on, causing it to catch on a rut and bend the jack out of shape.

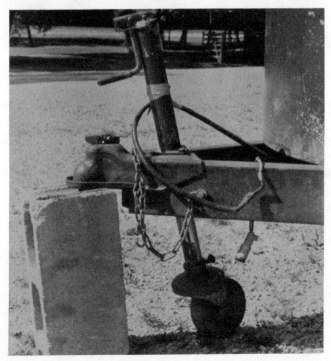

them working freely and to prevent binding rust. Grease the ball, its receptacle, and all hinge parts with wheel bearing grease to prevent metal bind when you're turning.

2. Wheel bearings and brakes should be inspected after the first five hundred miles of use and every two thousand miles thereafter.

3. Have tires rotated yearly.

4. If the trailer sits during the winter, or for months at other times of the year, either set it up on blocks or move it a couple of feet occasionally. Tires can develop a flat "set" to them when left in one spot.

5. Hose down floorboards after each haul to remove urine and manure wastes. These tend to rot the boards if left too long. Roll up floormats.

6. Have your trailer lights checked frequently and replace missing bulbs.

7. Carry steel wool with you and rub it over the light and brake plugs to remove corrosive deposits.

LOADING TECHNIQUES

Loading a horse puts him in a helpless and potentially dangerous situation. If you use patience and time as aids when schooling a horse to load, you can minimize his chances of being injured. A horse has a natural reaction to being crammed into a narrow, enclosed spot. His resistance to load is testimony to this fact.

Always allow yourself plenty of time to properly school to load, and do the same when you have to be somewhere at a certain time. Anticipate problems, have help available, block off avenues of escape, and give the horse hay once he's in the trailer. The horse will learn, in time, to obey you when you're firm about your desire to have him load, and are kind about asking.

Push-and-Pull Method

Attach a fifty-foot soft rope to the halter, run it forward through the trailer stall, and pass it through a tie loop at the front of the trailer. Then pass it out the side door and into the hands of the pulling assistant.

Next, attach a second rope to the tie loop on the rear channel of the trailer, next to the stall you're aiming for with the horse, and bring it around in back of the animal's rump (Figs. 170–174). As your pulling assistant urges from the front, you apply rump pressure.

Don't try to get the horse all the way in at first if he's really fighting. After a few steps, let the horse pause, but not too long. If his rump slides over the rope in his struggles, and the rear legs begin to fold, gently loosen the rope so he doesn't fall over backward.

217

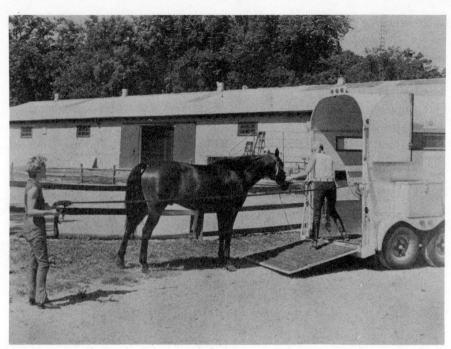

Figure 170. Load a balky horse by blocking his avenues of escape to the right and left.

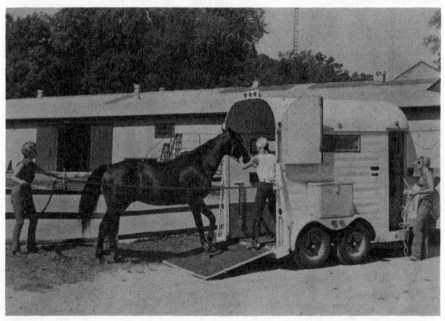

Figure 171. Gently move the rump strap in place and keep a firm hold on the lead line running through the front door of the trailer.

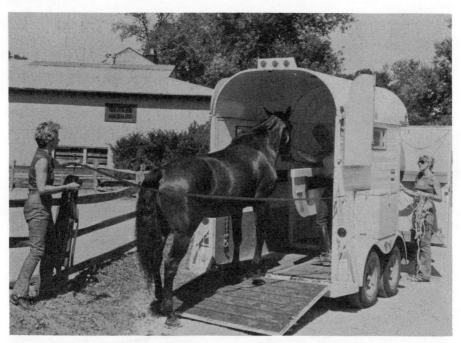

Figure 172. Give the horse time to size up the situation and avoid trying to rush him in.

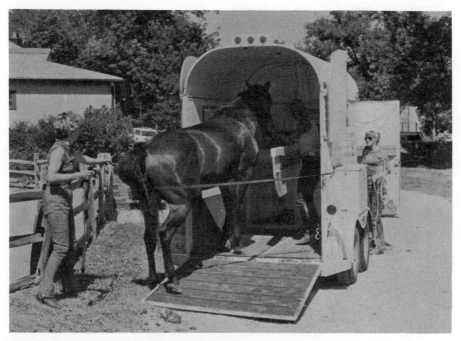

Figure 173. Everyone must move together to encourage the horse to enter, rather than avoid his destiny by stepping off the ramp.

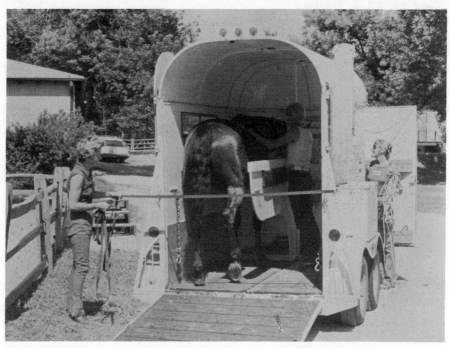

Figure 174. Once in the trailer, praise the horse and then get the ramp up quickly. Frequent repeats of this gentle method of loading will impress upon him that the procedure is harmless.

You can also employ the crop to the rump during this loading procedure, or snap the heels with a driving whip. Often this irritation will help the situation and clear the air.

Step-by-Step Method

Put one assistant on the pull rope and line up some others to help lift each foot and walk the horse in. This method is helpful with youngsters, and may also be employed along with the push-and-pull method.

The War Bridle

Following the directions in Figures 175–178, fashion a war bridle and work with the horse on the ground a few minutes to teach him to respond to the poll and jaw pressure. After each tug on it, loosen the bridle when the horse responds with a step forward.

Don't pull on the rope. Just exert a firm resistance and let the horse do the pulling back. He'll soon learn that going forward decreases pressure. Only then can you ask the horse to enter the trailer. Once you're in, don't tie the horse with the war bridle; use a halter.

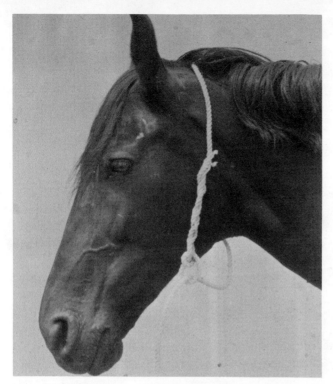

Figure 175. The first step in making a war bridle.

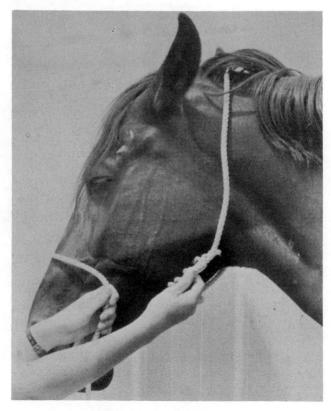

Figure 176. Step two.

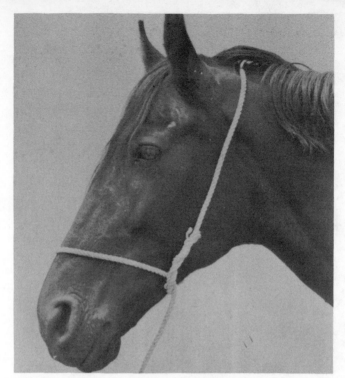

Figure 177. The third step is to pass the end of the line through the loop.

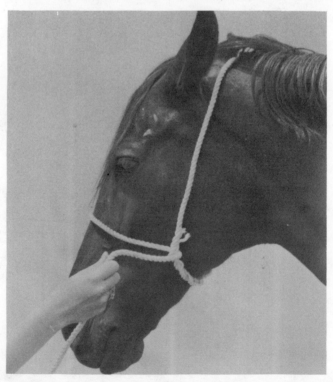

Figure 178. The last step is knowing how to pull the rope to put pressure on the poll and the jaws.

The Crop

Whether used to sharply smack the rump or flick the heels, the crop is a powerful persuader. It should be used sparingly, with small, light snaps instead of smashing blows. It's helpful to you only as long as the horse does not become terrified at the sight of it.

It is possible to load the horse by yourself with a long dressage whip by tapping the croup to indicate to the animal that you want a step forward. This method requires that you stay very near the side of your horse and keep your arm extended back all the while you load (Fig. 179). You'll find the method works better if you school the horse on the flat before asking him to walk into the trailer in response to the whip taps.

The Food Bribe

Many horsepersons achieve instant success in loading by bribing the horse with food. This method may work well with youngsters and hungry horses, but should not be used as a substitute to proper trailer training. Use it to take the fear out of the trailer, but don't connect it with a demand to enter. If you do, you might find yourself stranded at a show with a handful of carrots and a horse that has his feet firmly planted outside the trailer.

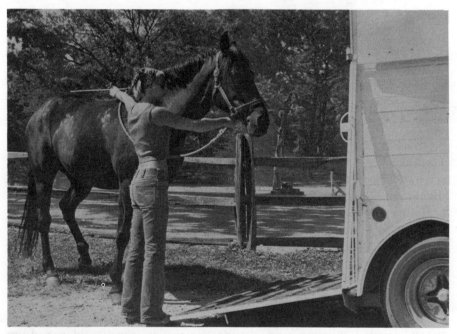

Figure 179. Many horses can be taught to walk right in the trailer by using the whip to tap their croup and stimulate a step.

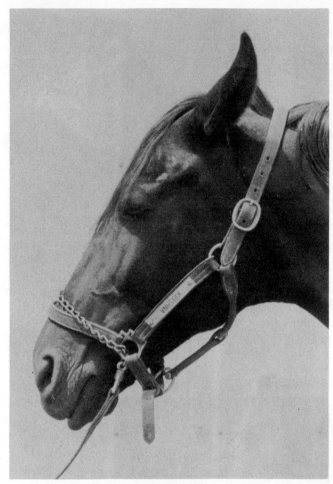

Figure 180. A nose chain should not be used unless all other methods fail. Be gentle in its use.

The Chain

The chain over the gums, through the mouth, or over the nose (Fig.180) should not be used unless you're very familiar with its dangers. It's a very brutal method of force, even when used with knowledge, and can cause the horse to rear and panic from the pain. There are many other methods that work better, and have fewer lingering aftereffects. Use patience, not force.

Sudden Surprises

When you're faced with a horse that has all his mental and physical energy devoted to remaining outside the trailer, the use of a sudden surprise can work wonders. A quick swat from a broom or a canvas

224

slapper on the rump will cause most horses to jump forward. If you supplement swats with encouraging clucks, the animals will get the association in time.

The Blindfold

Most stubborn fighters or truly panicked horses will become tractable when their eyes are covered. Use care when working with a blind horse, since the animal can step off the ramp or panic if frightened or hit. Fasten the blind so it can be quickly released, and don't employ the blindfold unless it's a last resort.

Grabbing the Tail

Gently taking the tail and pushing it over the back is helpful with youngsters. It allows the horse to be pushed along with little means to kick out or refuse. It's not recommended for use by a novice, since the tail can be damaged with excessive force.

Tranquilizers

Tranquilizers can be administered in oral granules or by injection. It's a humane method of calming a horse and smoothing over the loading procedure.

Tranquilizers are not generally employed as an everyday measure, but rather one for an emergency. The disadvantage to using one is that the horse may not be able to show due to the amount of the drug in his system. Ask your veterinarian or horse-show judge before trailering to a show under sedation.

Loading Hints

1. Never leave the horse alone in the trailer for long periods, or without supervision.

2. During insect season, fog the trailer for wasps and stinging insects. Use a fly sheet on the horse.

3. Always tie the horse with a quick release knot.

4. Don't tack up and load a horse that is not used to the procedure. It's a tight fit with a saddle on.

5. If the inside of your trailer is anything but white, paint it. Horses dislike dark interiors.

6. Sweep old manure from the stall before asking a horse to enter. Most of them object to stepping on it.

7. If possible, put on an easy loader first to give reassurance to a balky loader.

8. Close the front escape door when you load to dissuade the horse

from running over you and out the door. If you need added interior light, face the open end of the trailer toward the sun.

9. Always keep the hay net or manger full: food is a powerful reward for easy loading.

10. Wrap the legs and use a head bumper when you practice and haul.

11. Never attempt to hold onto the lead rope if the horse decides to exit quickly. This panics him and will cause him to raise his head and hit it on the roof.

Unloading

Many horses regard a torpedolike exit as the primary goal of their trailering experience, even when the tail chain is fastened. Such a style is both expensive and dangerous. There are though a few deterrents you may safely use to educate a horse to unload politely.

1. Take off the easily broken snaps on the tail chain and replace them with extra-large, heavy-duty hooks from the hardware store (Fig. 181). They won't give when the horse exits quickly. This should be done on all trailers regardless of the horse's temperament, since the hooks will hold in the event of an accident or struggle during transit.

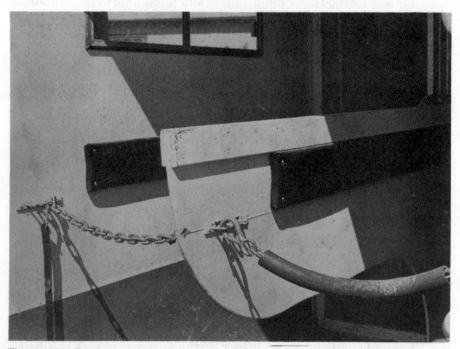

Figure 181. Replace standard latches with heavy-duty hooks purchased at a hardware store. These will not break if the horse struggles to back out of the trailer.

2. To keep the horse off the chain while towing, discourage hasty exits, and school the animal to slow down while departing, you can make and use an auxiliary rump strap of stirrup leather and filed down carpet tacks (Fig. 182). The strap is not used during hauls, just hooked up before you let down the ramp or open the doors.

3. You can slow down a fast ramp backer by parking your trailer close to the side of a building and dropping the ramp half a horse's length from the wall (with a step-down trailer there's usually not this problem). In the event you do have it with a step-down, utilize a full horse's length from the wall. When the horse shoots out from the trailer, he'll bounce his bottom off the wall.

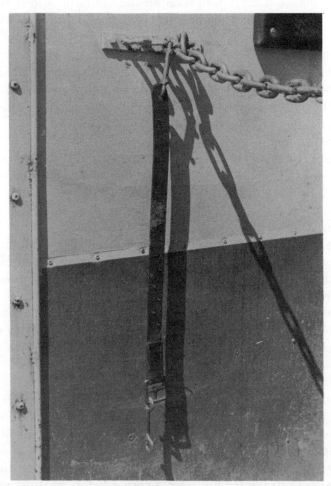

Figure 182. This homemade "antisit" strap is an old stirrup leather and filed down carpet tacks. It successfully dissuades a horse from backing too quickly during loading and unloading procedures.

4. If your horse backs crooked, have an assistant hold a longe line against the horse to help him back straight. You can also stand next to the horse and tap his side with a crop for direction.

HAULING TECHNIQUES

What makes a horse difficult to haul? In most cases it's a combination of a bad loading session and an even worse ride in the trailer. Once the horse associates the trailer confinement with being tossed from side to side, as the driver veers around the corner, or being slammed against the breast board or rump chain with each start and stop, he'll become a problem hauler. Reclaiming such an individual is a lot harder than practicing sensible, quiet loading techniques and slow driving habits.

Rearing
For the horse that rears in the trailer, try a tranquilizer to calm him down. Then tie his head with just a small amount of slack so he can't rear. If short tying causes panic, do the opposite: don't tie at all. If you can't get results with these methods, try a higher trailer and a good professional trainer.

Remember to always put on a head bumper and keep the hay net full for diversion. Often, the presence of a quiet companion in the trailer will lend a calming influence.

Pawing and Kicking
Pawing and kicking can occur because the trailer is too small, one horse doesn't like the other, the horse is high strung, lonesome, bored, frightened, or is anticipating being thrown around due to poor driving habits. The reasons are endless.

To protect his front legs, replace a solid front stall door with a breast bar, or put on knee guards and leg wraps. To deter injury to the horse being hauled with a kicker, use a full center partition.

Wall-Scrambling
One of the most dangerous horses to haul is the wall-scrambler, since he can cause the trailer to fishtail. The scrambler has been tossed around so many times he now uses the defense of leaning against the wall to brace himself against anticipated movement. The problem was originally caused by a thoughtless driver who took corners too fast, or didn't wait for the trailer to straighten out from a corner before putting on the gas.

You may never cure the horse of his fear, but you can help if you change the side he rides on, or put in a half divider to give him more room to spread his feet. These changes, coupled with correct driving habits, should eliminate some of the problem after the horse learns to relax.

It is not advised that you take out the partition in a two-horse trailer and let the horse ride without support. This is effective to a point, but dangerous in the event of an accident or swerving maneuver: the horse will go down.

Horses with balancing problems also sit on their chains or ride the ramp, along with scrambling up the sides of the trailer. Change your chain to a straight metal bar and start softening your starts and stops. If your driving is not at fault, your horse may need a longer stall to stop this habit.

Practice First

If you're not accustomed to trailering, practice first with an empty trailer. When you first haul loaded, expect a drag on your car from the horse's weight and try to slow down your starts, stops, and corners to accommodate the weight. As for accelerating, do it in slow motion. A jackrabbit start will put your trailer passengers back on the ramp or doors.

Don't ask for car speed until the momentum of your rig picks up. When you go into and come out of corners, try to keep the pace slow and constant. Accelerate *only* after your car and trailer are straightened out.

Reverse the procedure for stopping, i.e, keep the procedure slow and steady without sudden braking. If you use downshift #1 to help deceleration, be aware that the car might jerk. Practice before trying it with a load.

Road Hazards

Most other drivers on the road are unaware that you can't stop quickly with a trailer, nor can you get out of a tricky situation as they can. So try to avoid them, because they won't try to avoid you.

As you haul, you'll note that traffic pulls out in front of you without warning, often not bothering to speed up after they position themselves in your way. Turning without signaling is also a problem for you. Drivers change lanes, tailgate your trailer, and stop suddenly in front of you. You'll become more aware of these driving problems as you haul.

Your three defenses against traffic are your horn, lights, and a good defensive driving technique. This means to anticipate the worst and prepare for it. It helps to drive with your lights on to get the attention of other drivers, especially those who suddenly appear at a crossroad and appear not to know you're bearing down on them. When you drive defensively, try to establish eye contact with oncoming or turning drivers, or at least notice where the other driver is looking so you'll have an indication of where he's going or what he's going to do.

Make a practice of slowing down over bumps, gravel, and slick roads. These are road conditions that cause oscillation of the trailer and knock the horse around. Should fishtailing occur, there are three ways of handling it. You can (1) speed up and hope the trailer comes out of the sway, (2) begin to ease off the gas and apply gentle brake pressure *only* when the trailer swings back directly in line with the car, or (3) turn the wheel slightly in the direction of the sway until the situation corrects itself. *Never* apply the brakes to stop the vehicle, since you could cause the trailer to jackknife and possibly roll.

Hauling Tips

1. If you haul in an open trailer, use goggles to protect the horse's eyes against foreign objec's and dust.

2. Park in the shade if you must let your horse stand in the trailer.

3. Give an hour before and after hauling before you feed.

4. Spread straw or shavings over the trailer mat to encourage urination while trailering.

5. Don't haul young or green horses long distances until they have enough short trips to teach them balance.

6. After four hours of hauling, unload and give a half hour of exercise and rest. Don't haul longer than eight hours a day maximum.

7. Bring several days' supply of water from home, since most horses refuse to drink strange water.

8. It's better to trailer a horse too cool than too hot, so watch blanketing.

9. Never close up the trailer completely, since it becomes too hot and stuffy. In inclement weather, leave the vent open if you must close up the back and sides.

10. Remove shoes before a very long haul, since it allows better expansion and contraction of the feet.

11. Always haul a single horse on the left side. The road is built higher in the center to allow water drainoff to the sides, so the trailer will be more balanced this way.

12. When driving in the city with an electric brake control, turn down the juice so the constant stops and starts won't be as jerky.

13. Take off the jack wheel before hauling to avoid catching it on uneven terrain.

14. Always check the hookup before departing. Be sure the couple latch is secure and the ball tight within the receptacle. The chains should be attached, along with the breakaway wire, the brake and light plug working, and the brake control turned on.

15. Wrap the tail for horses that sit on the gate or are too long for the stall length.

16. On long trips, the use of a one-inch or less foam rubber pad (the same size as the mat), placed under the mat, will ease vibration and soreness.

Index